Current Topics in Environmental Health and Preventive Medicine

Series Editor

Takemi Otsuki
Kurashiki, Japan

Current Topics in Environmental Health and Preventive Medicine, published in partnership with the Japanese Society of Hygiene, is designed to deliver well written volumes authored by experts from around the globe, covering the prevention and environmental health related to medical, biological, molecular biological, genetic, physical, psychosocial, chemical, and other environmental factors. The series will be a valuable resource to both new and established researchers, as well as students who are seeking comprehensive information on environmental health and health promotion.

More information about this series at http://www.springer.com/series/13556

Masakazu Washio • Chikako Kiyohara

Editors

Health Issues and Care System for the Elderly

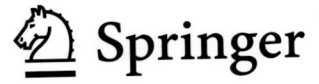 Springer

Editors
Masakazu Washio
St. Mary's College
Kurume
Fukuoka
Japan

Chikako Kiyohara
Department of Preventive Medicine
Kyushu University
Graduate School of Medicine
Higashi-ku
Fukuoka
Japan

ISSN 2364-8333   ISSN 2364-8341   (electronic)
Current Topics in Environmental Health and Preventive Medicine
ISBN 978-981-13-4678-1   ISBN 978-981-13-1762-0   (eBook)
https://doi.org/10.1007/978-981-13-1762-0

This Springer imprint is published by the registered company Springer Nature Singapore Pte Ltd.
The registered company address is: 152 Beach Road, #21-01/04 Gateway East, Singapore 189721, Singapore

Preface

In Japan, the population is aging, due to an increasing number of older people living longer and a decreasing birthrate. Improvements in public health and advances in medicine since World War II have given Japan one of the highest life expectancies in the world. However, increased life expectancy means that there will be more older people with chronic physical and mental illnesses, increasing the number of older people who need care in their daily living activities, as well as medical care for their chronic diseases. Therefore, the health problems of the elderly are an important issue in Japan. The rapidity of population aging in Japan is striking; it has taken only 24 years for the proportion of older people in the population to increase from 7% to 14%. The period during which the proportion of older people increased from 7% to 14% was much shorter in Japan than in western countries, and the period during which the proportion of older people has increased in other East Asian countries is also estimated to be much shorter than that in western countries.. Population aging has increased the costs of health care and social care for older people. Since non-communicable diseases, such as cardiovascular diseases and diabetes mellitus, in the middle-aged and the elderly have become new health problems in middle-income countries and in big cities in developing countries, the experience of Japan may give readers in other non-western countries useful information about how to cope with population aging. In this book, we would like to introduce the experience of Japan and discuss the public health problems of an aging society.

Kurume, Japan
Fukuoka, Japan

Masakazu Washio
Chikako Kiyohara

Contents

Chapter 1
Population Aging and Health of Older People in Japan: Introduction of Health Issues and Care System for the Elderly

Ikuko Miyabayashi, Masakazu Washio, Tomoko Yanagimoto, Eric Fortin, and Seiji Yasumura

Abstract Population aging is due to the increased number of older people living longer as well as the decreased birthrate. The improvement of public health and advances in medicine after World War II have given Japan one of the highest life expectancies in the world, while the emancipation of women following World War II has increased opportunities for higher education and gainful employment outside of the home, which may lead to advancing of late marriages and late birth and may influence the lower birthrate in Japan. Population aging has increased the costs of health and social care for older people, which have led to an interest in how to promote health in older people as well as how to define successful aging. Since the Confucian norm is shared among Japan and other East Asian countries, the experience of Japan may give readers useful information about how to cope with the population aging in other non-Western countries. In this chapter, we would like to introduce the experience of Japan and consider the public health problems in the aging society.

I. Miyabayashi
School of Nursing, Fukuoka University, Fukuoka City, Fukuoka, Japan

M. Washio (✉)
Department of Community Health and Clinical Epidemiology, St. Mary's College,
Kurume City, Fukuoka, Japan
e-mail: washiomasa@yahoo.co.jp

T. Yanagimoto
Advanced Midwifery Course, St. Mary's College, Kurume City, Fukuoka, Japan

E. Fortin
Department of Languages and Culture, St. Mary's College,
Kurume City, Fukuoka, Japan

S. Yasumura
Department of Public Health, Fukushima Medical University School of Medicine,
Fukushima City, Fukushima, Japan

© Springer Nature Singapore Pte Ltd. 2019
M. Washio, C. Kiyohara (eds.), *Health Issues and Care System for the Elderly*,
Current Topics in Environmental Health and Preventive Medicine,
https://doi.org/10.1007/978-981-13-1762-0_1

Keywords Population aging · Declining birthrate · Health problems · Successful aging · Confucian norm

1.1 Introduction

Decline in death rates and fertility have resulted in population aging [1]. Improvement of public health and advances in medicine after World War II have increased life expectancy as well as costs of health and social care for older people in Japan, which have led to an interest in how to promote health in older people as well as how to define successful aging.

Concepts of aging vary across societies and settings. In the past, the United Nations and other international agencies defined "older people" as 60 years and over, but recently there is a growing consensus that "older people" are persons who are 65 years old and over [1]. However, older people are not homogeneous, but very heterogeneous [1]. Some senior citizens are very frail and need care in their daily lives, while others play an active part in society, enjoy healthy retirement, or care for disabled relatives. The distinction between successful and usual aging was first raised by Rowe and Kahn [2]. Older people with successful aging are those without overt disease and who remain essentially independent until they experience a suddenly apparently natural death, while older people with usual aging are those who suffer from potentially preventable serious chronic diseases resulting in frailty and dependency. Their model of successful aging includes the following three components: (1) to prevent diseases and disabilities, (2) to maintain high physical and cognitive capacity, and (3) to continue social and productive activities in one's daily life [2]. In their model, only older people with high levels of function in these three components are considered to be aging "successfully," and this group may include only a small part of old-older people (80 years and over).

On the other hand, Baltes PB and Baltes MM proposed an alternative model [3]. In Baltes' model, the personal experience of aging is subjective and unique, and each person can remain mentally strong in spite of disability or frailty and can adapt to limitations as the result of one's own aging [3–5]. A personal opinion on one's health as well as one's health status varies between individuals in the elderly population. Therefore, it is important to recognize this heterogeneity when we define their needs, offer health and welfare services for senior citizens, and make a health plan for the future.

Population aging is not only due to the increased number of older people living longer but also due to the decreased birthrate, leading to a decline in young people [1]. In addition, the falling birthrate decreases the future population in the long term [1]. In this chapter, we would like to introduce the phenomenon of population aging in Japan and consider the public health problems in the aging society.

1.2 Population Aging in Japan: Demographics, Projections, and Causes

Before World War II, the average life expectancy at birth was shorter than 50 years in Japan (i.e., 46.9 years for men and 49.6 years for women in 1935–1936) (Table 1.1) [6]. However, improvement of public health and advances in medicine after World War II has given Japan one of the highest average life expectancies at birth in the world (i.e., 80.8 years for men and 87.0 years for women in 2015) (Table 1.1) [7]. On the other hand, the live birthrate (per every 1000 Japanese people) decreased from 28.1 in 1950 to 8.0 in 2015 (Table 1.2) [7]. Similarly, total fertility rate, gross reproduction rate, and net reproduction rate decreased from 3.65, 1.77, and 1.50 in 1950 to 1.45, 0.71, and 0.70 in 2015 (Table 1.2) [7].

The emancipation of women from Japanese household legal structure after World War II gives Japanese women an increased opportunity for higher education, gainful employment outside of home, and later age at marriage (i.e., advancing of late marriages). Age at first marriage of women increased from 23.0 years old in 1950 to 29.4 years old in 2015 [8, 9], which is one of the latest ages at first marriage in the

Table 1.1 Trend in life expectancy at birth in Japan

Year	Males (year)	Females (year)
1891–1898	42.80	44.30
1899–1903	43.97	44.85
1909–1913	44.25	44.73
1921–1925	42.06	43.20
1926–1930	44.82	46.54
1935–1936	46.92	49.63
1947	50.06	53.96
1950–1952	59.57	62.97
1955	63.60	67.75
1960	65.32	70.19
1965	67.74	72.92
1970	69.31	74.66
1975	71.73	76.89
1980	73.35	78.76
1985	74.78	80.48
1990	75.92	81.90
1995	76.38	82.85
2000	77.72	84.64
2005	78.56	85.52
2010	79.55	86.30
2015	80.75	86.99

Source: Trend of national health 1976, Trend of national health 2017–2018

Table 1.2 Trend in live birthrates, total fertility rates, and reproduction rates in Japan

Year	Live birthrate (per 1000)	Total fertility rate	Gross reproduction rate	Net reproduction rate
1950	28.1	3.65	1.77	1.50
1960	17.2	2.00	0.95	0.92
1970	18.8	2.13	1.03	1.00
1980	13.6	1.75	0.85	0.83
1990	10.0	1.54	0.75	0.74
2000	9.5	1.36	0.66	0.65
2010	8.5	1.39	0.67	0.67
2015	8.0	1.45	0.71	0.70

Source: Trend of national health 2017–2018

world. Late age at first marriage (i.e., 29.4 years old for women and 31.1 years old for men [9]) may shorten the reproductive span of married couples in Japan [8]. Furthermore, the proportion of never-married Japanese women at age 50 (i.e., the rate of never-married women in their reproductive span) increased from 1.4% in 1950 to 14.1% in 2015 [9, 10]. Since much fewer children are born out of marriage in Japan (2.1%) than in Western countries (France 52.6%, the UK 43.7%, Sweden 54.7%, Germany 32.7%, the USA 40.6%) [11], the increase in the rate of never-married women may contribute to the drop of birthrate in Japan. Therefore, we should provide social systems in which young married couples can bring up their children without a heavy burden so that young couples can marry at an early age.

On the other hand, industrialization, urbanization, and social mobility after World War II influenced Japanese family structure. The proportion of three-generation family households decreased from 19.2% in 1970 [12] to 5.9% in 2016 [7], while the proportion of nuclear family households (i.e., married couples, parents and children, a parent and children) increased from 45.4% in 1955 [12] to 60.5% in 2016 [7]. Most young Japanese women care for their infants and children without any help of their mothers or mothers-in-law in their households, which may cause some young mothers to refrain from having further children.

According to a 2010 report of the National Institute of Population and Social Security Research, over 80% of Japanese married couples have two or fewer children (i.e., 13.6% have no child, 22.3% have one child, and 45.6% have two children), while only 17.7% of married couples have three or more children (i.e., 15.7% have three children, 1.7% have four children, and 0.3% have five or more children) [11]. One-third of first married Japanese couples have smaller numbers of children than the desired number of children they would like to have [11], and about 60% of them answer that they do so because of expensive child-raising and child-education costs [11]. When young couples, who do not live with their mothers/mothers-in-law, cannot leave their child with a licensed nursery school, most young Japanese women are obliged to decide whether they stop working to care for their child or leave their child with a costly unauthorized nursery school.

The combination of the increased life expectancy (i.e., decreased age-adjusted death rate) and decreased reproduction rate has brought an increase in the proportion

Table 1.3 Trends in population structure in Japan

	Population composition by major group (%)			Dependency ratio			Elderly to children ratio
Year	0–14 years old	15–64 years old	65+ years old	Total dependency ratio	Children dependency ratio	Old-age dependency ratio	
1930	36.6	58.7	4.8	70.5	62.4	8.1	13
1940	36.1	59.2	4.7	69.0	61.0	8.0	13
1950	35.4	59.6	4.9	67.7	59.4	8.3	14
1960	30.2	64.1	5.7	55.9	47.0	8.9	19
1970	24.0	68.9	7.1	45.1	34.9	10.3	29
1980	23.5	67.4	9.1	48.4	34.9	13.5	39
1990	18.2	69.7	12.1	43.5	26.2	17.3	66
2000	14.6	68.1	17.4	46.9	21.4	25.5	119
2010	13.2	63.8	23.0	56.8	20.7	36.1	174
2015	12.6	60.7	26.6	64.7	20.8	43.9	211

Source: Trend of national health 1998 [12], Trend of national health 2017–2018 [7]
Note: Total dependency ratio = (children population + aged population)/working age population
Children dependency ratio = children population/working age population
Old-age dependency ratio = aged population/working age population

of older people (i.e., 65 years and over) in Japan, where the proportion of older people increased from 4.9% in 1950 to 26.6% in 2015 (Table 1.3) [7]. As shown in Table 1.3, the old-age dependency ratio increased from 8.3 in 1950 to 43.9 in 2015 [7]. According to the medium variant projections of the National Institute of Population and Social Security Research, the population of Japan is estimated to decrease from 127 million in 2015 to 88 million in 2065 [13].

The public pension system for senior citizens is operated with the premium burden on the working generation [10]. In 2015, 40 million Japanese people (i.e., 30% of the population) receive public pension, which accounts for 70% of the income of the elderly households in Japan [10]. In this system, working generations do not store funds for themselves in the future, but support older people living in the same time period. This system can avoid loss of funds due to price listing in future [10]. However, the revision of the system will be needed in order to adapt the advanced aging society to the falling birthrate and declining population.

1.3 Measures to the Declining Labor Force

1.3.1 Population Aging and the Labor Force

Although the labor force population increased from 51.53 million in 1970 to 65.98 million in 2015 [14], it is estimated that the total population will decrease from 127 million in 2015 to 88 million in 2065 due to the lower birthrate in Japan [13].

Because population aging associated with declining population will result in a decreased labor force population, securing the labor force is important for Japan to maintain its national strength.

1.3.2 Support for Women Not to Lose Gainful Employment Outside of the Home After the Delivery

In 2016, 25.3 million women work outside of the home and are 44.2% of total employees in Japan [10]. However, there are still many young women who stopped working outside of the home in order to care for their child because of the shortage of nursery schools. Nearly half of women (47%) lost gainful employment outside of the home after the delivery of their first child in 2010–2014 [10]. In order to support young women so that they can keep working outside of the home even after delivery, the Japanese government promotes the "Plan for accelerated elimination of children on waiting lists to get in nursery schools" [10, 15], which may also help young couples to marry at a younger age as well as to have additional children in their families (i.e., increase the birthrate in Japan).

1.3.3 Ensuring Employment Until Age 65 and Supporting Reemployment

In order to ensure employment until age 65, the Japanese government settled a law to oblige the companies to employ all applicants until age 65. In 2015, 99.2% of companies with 31 workers or more provided either of the following three measures: (1) raising of the retirement age to age 65, (2) introduction of a continued employment system, or (3) abolition of a retirement age [14]. In addition, 54.4% of companies provided a continued employment system for those 65 years old and over, 15.5% of companies raised the retirement age to 65 and over, and 2.6% of companies abolished their retirement age [14].

Among 35,000 workers who wanted to work after the retirement age, 82.1% were continuously hired after the retirement age of 65 [14]. However, there were only 20.1% of older workers who continued to be hired until the age 70 and over [14].

Since older people are not homogeneous but very heterogeneous [1], reemployment for work that matches personal experience and remaining capacity seems to be important for older people so that they can adapt to limitations as the result of their own aging [3–5]. In 2015, 74.4% of older workers aged 65 and over were non-regular employment workers [14]. The reason why they work as non-regular employment workers was because (1) they wanted to work at their convenient time (31.7%), (2) they wanted to receive a household subsidy or tuition (20.1%), (3) they wanted to use their professional skills (14.9%), (4) they had no chance to obtain a regular employment job (8.8%), (5) they wanted shorter commuting time (i.e., the workplaces near to home) (4.0%), or (6) they wanted to balance work with housework, childcare, or elderly care (3.2%) [14].

In 2016, the Japanese government revised a law in order to support older persons who want to continue working at the age of 65 and over [14]. The aims of the law are (1) to maintain the working environment which support older people to continue working without anxiety and (2) to target newly hired older workers at the age of 65 and over for employment insurance [14]. Since older people are not homogeneous but very heterogeneous [1], reemployment for work that matches personal experience and remaining capacity seems to be important so that older people adapt to limitations due to aging and undergo successful aging [3–5].

1.3.4 Health Promotion and Prevention of Chronic Disease for Working Ages

Our health status in the later life is influenced by our life experiences throughout life. Therefore, health promotion and prevention of chronic diseases during the working years are important to prevent a decline in the labor force as well as to obtain healthy aging.

In 1978, the Ministry of Health and Welfare (currently the Ministry of Health, Labour and Welfare) started the first phase of Japan's national plan for health which focused on secondary prevention at working ages (e.g., health checkup, screening for cancer) [16]. In 1988, the second phase of Japan's national plan for health began, which included secondary prevention as well as health promotion (e.g., health education to prevent lifestyle-related diseases) [16].

In 2000, the Ministry of Health and Welfare (currently the Ministry of Health, Labour and Welfare) announced a new approach campaign called "Healthy Japan 21" (i.e., the third phase of Japan's national plan for health) to promote better health of each citizen who will live in Japan in the twenty-first century [16], which covers specific areas in lifestyles and lifestyle-related diseases (e.g., tobacco smoking, alcohol drinking, nutrition and dietary habits, leisure time physical activity and exercise, rest, dental and oral health, obesity and diabetes, stroke and ischemic heart disease, cancer) [16].

Targets for "Healthy Japan 21" include the prevention of lifestyle-related diseases (e.g., cancer, stroke and ischemic heart disease, diabetes, chronic obstructive lung disease) as well as the maintenance of functions necessary for engaging in social life (e.g., mental health) [16].

1.4   Health Problems of Older People

1.4.1   High Prevalence of Chronic Disease and Multiple Diagnoses

Aging increases chronic diseases in the elderly. More than half of older people (65 years and over) who live in the community attend hospitals as outpatients in Japan (68.2% for men and 69.1% for women), and the proportion of those who attend hospitals increased in old-older people (75 years and over) (72.5% for men and 73.0% for women), which is greater than the proportion of those who attend hospitals among the general population (i.e., 37.2% for men and 40.7% for women) [7].

Multiple diagnoses are common in older persons, which may be explained in by the following ways [17]. First, common disorders (e.g., hypertension, osteoarthritis, diabetes mellitus, vascular disease, and dementia) increase with aging [17]. Second, disturbance of the immune system as well as lifelong exposure to carcinogens during their long lifetime brings an increased risk of cancer [17]. Third, compared with young- or middle-aged persons, an illness (e.g., respiratory infection) affecting one system is more likely to lead to disorders in another in the elderly [17]. Fourth, a vascular event (e.g., stroke) may develop at any time in older people although vascular diseases may develop gradually [17]. Last, immobility associated with neurological or musculoskeletal disorders may increase the risk of complications such as falls, deep vein thrombosis, and pulmonary embolism [17].

Therefore, it is important for older people to prevent an acute illness which may worsen underlying chronic diseases. The Japanese Ministry of Health, Labour and Welfare recommends influenza vaccinations for older people [7]. In Japan, older people (i.e., 65 years old and over) have been subsidized by their municipality since 2001 for influenza vaccination under the Preventive Vaccination Law. The aim of influenza vaccination is not only to prevent the development of influenza infection but also to prevent severe complications following influenza infection (e.g., pneumonia, heart failure, stroke, falls, and death) [7]. Ozasa et al. [18] reported that influenza vaccination was effective for high fever (i.e., 38.0 °C and over) during the influenza season among the non-institutionalized Japanese elderly population (OR = 0.77, 95% confidence interval: 0.40–1.47). On the other hand, Washio et al. [19] reported that influenza vaccination reduced the risk of pneumonia acquired outside hospitals among the Japanese elderly during the winter months (OR = 0.33, 95% confidence interval: 0.13–0.90).

1.4.2   Hypoalbuminemia and Frailty

Population aging increases not only the elderly with chronic diseases but also the elderly with decreased mental and physical function, which brings increase in older people who need care [20]. Therefore, in 2017, the Japanese Ministry of Health,

Labour and Welfare announced a new health-care approach for the elderly called "Tentative Health business guidelines on the basis of characteristics of elderly persons" in order to prevent the aggravation of chronic diseases as well as to prevent a decrease in the mental and physical function in older people [20].

The prevalence of hypoalbuminemia is reported to increase with age in Japanese elderly [21, 22], and Kitamura et al. [23] reported an inverse causal association between serum albumin and activities of daily living (ADL) among senior citizens with frailty in Japan. Hypoalbuminemia increases the risk of the development of pneumonia in Japanese elderly (OR = 9.25, 95% CI = 4.04–21.14), while an impaired ability to perform one's daily living (i.e., ADL without limitation) reduces the risk of pneumonia in the elderly (OR = 0.34, 95% CI = 0.12–0.80) [19]. Pneumonia is the third leading cause of death among Japanese elderly (65 years old and older) [7]. Therefore, public health services directed toward maintaining nutritional status and ability to carry out ADL are helpful for the elderly to age successfully.

1.4.3 Prevalence and Number of Dementia Among the Older People in Japan

Dementia presents with a progressive loss of cognitive function from any of several domains (e.g., memory impairment, language deficits, disinhibition, deficits in executive function, sleep disorders, hallucinations) [24, 25]. Among the neurodegenerative dementia, Alzheimer's disease (AD), dementia with Lewy bodies (DLB), frontotemporal lobular degeneration dementia (FTLD), and dementia in Parkinson's disease predominate with aging [24, 25]. Cerebrovascular disease, which may cause vascular dementia (VaD), may coexist with neurodegenerative dementia [24, 25].

In Japan, the prevalence of dementia is estimated to be 15% (95% confidence intervals: 12–17%) among the older people (65 years old and over), and the number of older persons with dementia is estimated to be 4,390,000 persons (95% confidence intervals: 3,500,000–4,970,000) in 2010 [26, 27]. Among them, 2.8 million older persons with dementia used care services (e.g., home visiting nursing service) under the public long-term care insurance system (LTCIS) for the elderly [26, 27]. In 2015, the Japanese government made a new national plan in order to support the older persons with dementia and their family caregivers as well as to prevent the development and progression of dementia [7].

In an ecological study by Shigeta [28], there was a positive association between the year of the survey and the ratio of the prevalence of AD to that of VaD, and the prevalence of AD shows a positive relation to the year of the survey. The findings of this ecological study may suggest that the number of AD patients increased with the number of older persons with dementia although the number of VaD patients did not increase according to the increase in the number of older person because of the prevention of cerebrovascular diseases with blood pressure control through various public health activities (e.g., lifestyle modification including weight control, exercise, and diet [29]) or drug treatment such as antihypertensive agents.

Dementia symptoms may also occur in psychiatric disorders other than dementia (e.g., anxiety, depression), metabolic disorders, infections, autoimmune disorders, nutritional disorders, pharmaceutical drug effects, or normal-pressure hydrocephalus [25]. Although these conditions may be treatable in the early phase, dementia symptoms will become irreversible dementia if these conditions persist long. Therefore, education for health-care workers to distinguish "treatable dementia" from dementia as well as education for citizens to reduce risk of VaD (e.g., prevention and control of VaD risk factors such as hypertension [30]) is important to reduce the development of dementia other than neurodegenerative dementia.

On the other hand, maintaining an active life is believed to be effective for senior citizens to preserve their physical and mental health [31]. An active and social integrated lifestyle in later life is suggested to protect against dementia including AD [31].

Cerebrovascular disease ranks as one of the major causes of death in industrialized countries (e.g., the fourth major cause of death in Japan [7]), and it is also a major contributor of disability [32]. Therefore, the prevention of cerebrovascular disease as well as the early rehabilitation for patients with cerebrovascular disease to reduce their disabilities is important to prevent dementia among older people.

1.5   Speed of Population Aging

Table 1.4 illustrates international comparison of the speed of population aging among selected countries in Europe, North America, and East Asia with respect to the year that they either attained or expected to attain from 7% to 14% level in terms

Table 1.4 Speed of population aging in selected countries

Country	Years attaining the specified percentage of older people (65 years old and older) among the total population		Years required to increase the proportion of older people from 7% to 14%
	7%	14%	
Japan	1970	1994	24
South Korea	1999	2017	18
Taiwan	1995	2020	25
China	2002	2025	23
Singapore	2000	2020	20
Thailand	2010	2030	20
Germany	1932	1972	40
U K	1929	1975	46
USA	1942	2014	72
Sweden	1887	1972	85
France	1864	1979	115

Source: White paper (Japanese Ministry of Health, Labour and Welfare), 2016 [14]
Wakabayashi K. Aziya Kenkyu (Asian Studies), 2006 [33]

of the population of the older people (65 years old and over) [14], [33]. The rapidity of population aging in East Asia is very impressive [14, 33]. It took only 24 years in Japan for the proportion of older people to increase from 7% to 14% [14]. On the other hand, compared with Japan, the period of doubling of the proportion of older people (i.e., from 7% to 14%) is longer in the Western countries (e.g., France 115 years, the UK 46 years, and the USA 69 years) [14]. On the other hand, it was estimated to take 23 years in China and 20 years in Singapore for the proportion of older people to increase from 7% to 14% [14, 33].

In a country, where social security programs have been scarce and care for the elderly has largely depended on the family, it remains a question whether younger generations will be able to take care of the increasing elderly population [34]. In China, a young married couple has to take care of four old parents because of the one-child policy [34]. Although nations are different between Japan and other East Asian countries, the Confucian norm of frail piety (i.e., ancestor worship and respect for the elderly) is shared among East Asian countries [34].

Since a rapidly progressing population aging gives a greater impact on society and economy than slowly progressing one, the experience of Japan may provide readers useful information about how to face the population aging in other Asian countries with the rapidly progressing population aging.

1.6 Discussion

Aging is a lifelong process and continues throughout life, and for each person, our health status in later life is influenced by our different life experiences throughout life. The functional capacity of our biological systems increases during the first years in life, reaches its peak in early adulthood, and naturally declines thereafter [35]. The prevention of diseases and disabilities is closely related with maintenance of high physical and cognitive capacity and continuation of social and productive activities in our later life. The model of successful aging proposed by Rowe and Kahn [2] includes all of these three components.

In a large scale of prospective cohort study in Taiwan [36], five lifestyle risk factors (i.e., smoking, alcohol consumption, insufficient fruit/vegetable intake, insufficient physical activity, and non-ideal body mass index) are responsible for 25 % of cancer incidence and 40% of cancer death, while two chronic diseases/markers (i.e., cardiovascular disease and chronic kidney disease) are responsible for 20% of cancer incidence and 40% of cancer death.

"Healthy Japan 21" focuses on the importance of primary prevention because lifestyle factors are related to development and progression of chronic diseases [16]. With respect to tobacco smoking, "Healthy Japan 21" decreased the rates of current smokers (i.e., adults who have smoking habits) from 47.4% for men and 11.5% for women in 2000 to 30.1% for men and 9.7% for women in 2016 [7]. Since tobacco smoking increases the risk of chronic diseases (e.g., cancers, stroke, ischemic heart disease, chronic obstructive lung disease, and type 2 diabetes) [7], it is very important to reduce the rate of current smokers as well as to avoid the exposure of tobacco smoke for nonsmokers. In addition, secondary prevention (e.g., health checkups and screening for cancer) and tertiary prevention (e.g., rehabilitation for patients with stroke, ischemic heart disease, or lung disease) are also important to prevent decline in labor force as well as to achieve successful aging in the later life.

Population aging is caused by the combination of increased life expectancy (i.e., decreased death rate in young- and middle-aged people) and decreased birthrate, and the dropped birthrate decreases future population in the long term [1]. Conditions, such as an increase in the number of unmarried people and late marriages may have a direct impact in creating low fertility. On the other hand, there are many young couples who hesitate to have another child because of expensive child-raising and child's education costs. If there is neither a licensed nursery school for their child nor a family member who can care for their child (e.g., their mother), young women may lose gainful employments outside of the home after delivery, due to the fact they must care for their child, as women are assumed to be the main source of support for family members in Japan [37]. Otherwise, they are obliged to pay high expenses for leaving their child with an unauthorized nursery school. However, nearly half of women (47%) lost gainful employment outside of the home after delivery of the first child in 2010–2014 [10]. Therefore, benefit-in-kind (e.g., nursery school, day-care center for children, baby-sitter, accommodation postpartum care, grandmother/grandmother-in-law in the same household) seem to be more helpful than cash-benefit for young women to maintain their gainful employments outside of the home after delivery. In order to weaken the negative impact of the rapid population aging in Japan, we should provide enough numerical licensed nursery schools and other childcare services for young couples and their children. In addition to these social services, we should provide effective education programs from a primary school in order to create a new culture in which both fathers and mothers participate in child-rearing because the participation of fathers in child-rearing is still smaller in Japan than in Western countries [11, 38].

With respect to the child's education, Japanese parents spend much more money on university education than primary school and secondary school education, which may influence the number of children in young couples, because they must save money not only for their own living expenses of the old age but also for their child's university education. The Ministry of Education, Culture, Sports, Science and Technology estimates that educational expenses account for half of the averaging disposal income of the workers in a family of parents and two children when both children go to private university [39]. Furthermore, when two children room and board at a private university, educational expenses account for 80% of the averaging disposal income of the worker [39].

Although many university students receive scholarships, most funds are obtained through loans with a return duty, which may influence marriage at a late age among university graduates. In order to reduce the marriage at late age among university graduates, it may be time to discuss whether Japan should make the tuition of national universities free or increase the number of university students who receive scholarships without the return duty regardless of household income.

Population aging is associated with declining population. It is estimated that the total population will decrease from 127 million in 2015 to 88 million in 2065 [13]. There are some efforts to minimize the negative impact of the population decline on economic activities in Japan. First, the Japanese government promotes the "Plan for accelerated elimination of children on waiting lists to get in nursery schools" so that young women can keep working outside of the home even after delivery [10, 15]. The women' labor force participation rate is tending to increase in Japan. Dividing the labor force by age-group, the transition showed an M-shaped curve in the 1970s, with the age bracket of 25–34 being the bottom, suggesting that women tend to terminate the employment during the periods of childcare [40]. Recently, however, an M-shaped curve is changing to a reverse U-shaped curve, suggesting the increase in the proportion of women who continues working outside of the home all through their life [40].

Second, the Japanese government revised a law in order to support older persons who want to continue working at the age of 65 and over [14]. Third, the Japanese government announced a new national plan which covers specific areas in lifestyles and lifestyle-related diseases in order to prevent the development and progression of chronic diseases [16].

However, some recommends the acceptance of the foreign workers with a view to compensating for the shortage in our labor force. The technical intern training program was started in 1993, in order to transfer technical skills, techniques, and knowledge to developing countries, which is the system to accept the foreign workers in the short term, although it does not allow them to be permanent residents [41]. Although technical intern trainees have come to provide essential labors for Japan, they are not completely protected as employees under the Labor Standards Acts [41]. Since the declining young workers means decreased successors of traditional technologies, it may be time to choose whether to abandon some traditional skills and technologies or to accept foreign workers as successors of traditional skills and technologies. A review of the technical intern training program is necessary in order to work with foreign workers as permanent co-workers in Japan. When accepting foreign workers, the Japanese government should provide opportunities for their children to learn at elementary school and junior high school in Japan.

Although 2.8 million older Japanese with dementia used care services under the public long-term care insurance system (LTCIS) for the elderly in 2010 [26], population aging causes a shortage of labor for elderly care. When we ask foreign care workers or foreign nurses to care for the Japanese elderly, we should ask them to learn Japanese culture as well as Japanese language. At that time, we should enhance the educational system to support foreign candidates of care workers/nurses so that they can surely learn the minimum knowledge necessary for caring for Japanese elderly. First, we should teach students only important things and should not teach them too many things. Second, we should teach them in a way that they come to consider why they must act in certain ways when they care for Japanese elderly persons. Third, we should show them how they will be treated at their workplaces after their training when they care for Japanese elderly. It may be time to discuss about how we can provide an education system to support their study without having to bear a heavy financial burden in Japan.

The improvement of public health and advances in medicine after World War II reduced the death from infectious diseases, such as pulmonary tuberculosis, and increased life expectancy in Japan [7], while industrialization, urbanization, and social mobility after World War II influenced Japanese lifestyles and family structures. Westernized dietary habits (e.g., increased consumption of beef, pork, and butter) and decrease of physical activities due to car ownership and spread of electric household appliances (e.g., electric washing machine) may have increased the proportion of obesity, which brings an increased risk of death from lifestyle-related diseases (e.g., cancer, stroke, and ischemic heart disease). Therefore, "Healthy Japan 21" focuses on the importance of primary prevention of lifestyle-related diseases [16]. On the other hand, the emancipation of women from the traditional Japanese household legal structure and the decreased proportion of young couples who live with their mothers/mothers-in-law in the same households may influence the falling birthrate in Japan.

The rapidity of population aging in Japan is very impressive. It took only 24 years in Japan for the proportion of older people to increase from 7% to 14% [14]. Compared with Western countries, the period during which the proportion of older people had doubled was much shorter in Japan and is estimated to be much shorter in other East Asian countries as well. Since the Confucian norm is shared among Japan and other East Asian countries [34], the experience of Japan (i.e., both success experiences and failure experiences) may give readers useful information about how to cope with the population aging in other Asian countries.

References

1. Ebrahim S, Byles JE. Health of older people. In: Detels R, Beaglehole R, Langsang MA, Gulliford M, editors. Oxford textbook of public health. 5th ed. Oxford: Oxford University Press; 2009. p. 1496–514.
2. Rowe JW, Kahn RL. Human ageing: usual and successful. Science. 1987;237:143–9.
3. Baltes PB, Baltes MM. Psychological perspectives on successful aging: The model of selective optimization with compensation. In: Baltes PB, Baltes MM, editors. Successful aging: perspectives from the behavioral sciences. Cambridge: Cambridge University Press; 1990. p. 1–34.
4. Baltes MM, Carstensen LL. The process of successful ageing. Ageing Soc. 1996;i6: 397–422.
5. Donnellan C. The Baltes' model of successful aging and its considerations for aging life care™/geriatric care management. J Aging Life Care. Fall 2015. http://www.aginglifecare-journal.org/the-baltes-model-of-successful-aging-and-its-considerations-for-aging-life-care-geriatric-care-management/. Accessed 21 Feb 2018.
6. Health and Welfare Statistics Association. Trend of national health 1976. Tokyo: Health and Welfare Statistics Association; 1976. (in Japanese)
7. Health, Labour and Welfare Statistics Association. Trend of national health 2017–2018. Tokyo: Health, Labour and Welfare Statistics Association; 2017. (in Japanese)
8. Kono S. Demographic aspects of population ageing in Japan. In: Takagi F, editor. Aging in Japan 2003. Tokyo: Japan aging research center; 2003. p. 7–51.

9. Cabinet Office, Government of Japan. 2017 declining birth rate White Paper. (in Japanese). 2017. http://www8.cao.go.jp/shoushi/shoushika/whitepaper/measures/w-2017/29pdfgaiyoh/29gaiyoh.html. Accessed 22 Feb 2018.
10. Ministry of Health, Labour and Welfare. A 2017 White Paper; 2017 (in Japanese).
11. Cabinet Office, Government of Japan. (in Japanese) A 2014 Declining Birth Rate White Paper; 2014 (in Japanese). http://www8.cao.go.jp/shoushi/shoushika/whitepaper/measures/w-2014/26pdfgaiyoh/26gaiyoh.html. Accessed 22 Feb 2018.
12. Health and Welfare Statistics Association. Trend of national health 1998. Tokyo: Health and Welfare Statistics Association; 1998. (in Japanese)
13. Health, Labour and Welfare Statistics Association. Trend of national welfare and care 2017–2018. Tokyo: Health, Labour and Welfare Statistics Association; 2017. (in Japanese)
14. Ministry of Health, Labour and Welfare. 2016 White Paper; 2016 (in Japanese).
15. Ministry of Health, Labour and Welfare. Plan for accelerated elimination of children on waiting lists to get in nursery schools (in Japanese). 2013. www.mhlw.go.jp/bunya/kodomo/pdf/taikijidokaisho_01.pdf. Accessed 22 Feb 2018.
16. Health and Welfare Statistics Association (2004). Trend of national health 2004. Tokyo: Health and Welfare Statistics Association. (in Japanese).
17. Rai GS, Mulley GP. Clinical ageing. In: Rai GS, Mulley GP, editors. Elderly medicine, a training guide. London: Martin Dunitz; 2002. p. 15–7.
18. Ozasa K, Kawahito Y, Doi T, Watanabe Y, Washio M, Mori M, et al. Retrospective assessment of influenza vaccine effectiveness among the non-institutionalized elderly population in Japan. Vaccine. 2006;24:2537–43.
19. Washio M, Kondo K, Fujisawa N, Harada E, Tashiro H, Mizokami T, et al. Hypoalbuminemia, influenza vaccination and other factors related to the development of pneumonia acquired outside hospitals in southern Japan: a case-control study. Geriatr Gerontol Int. 2016;16(2):223–9.
20. Senior Citizen Medical Division, Health Insurance Bureau, Ministry of Health, Labour and Welfare. Tentative health business guidelines on the basis of characteristics of elderly persons. (in Japanese). 2017. http://www.mhlw.go.jp/file/06-Seisakujouhou-12400000-Hoken-kyoku/0000167494.pdf. Accessed 28 Mar 2018.
21. Gomi I, Fukushima H, Shiraki M, Miwa Y, Ando T, Takai K, et al. Relationship between serum albumin level and aging in community-dwelling self-reported elderly population. J Nutr Sci Vitaminol. 2007;53:37–42. https://doi.org/10.3177/jnsv.53.37.
22. Miyake M, Ogawa Y, Yoshida Y, Imaki M. Seven-year large cohort study for the association of serum albumin level and aging among community dwelling elderly. Seibutsu shiryou bunseki (J Anal Biosci). 2011;34(4):281–6.
23. Kitamura K, Nakamura K, Nishiwaki T, Ueno K, Nakazawa A, Hasegawa M. Determination of whether the association between serum albumin and activities of daily living in frail elderly people is causal. Environ Health Prev Med. 2012;17:164–8. https://doi.org/10.1007/s12199-011-0233-y.
24. Kukull WA, Bowen J. Neurologic diseases, epidemiology, and public health. In: Detels R, Beaglehole R, Langsang MA, Gulliford M, editors. Oxford textbook of public health. Oxford: Oxford University Press; 2009. p. 1132–59.
25. Bourgeois MS, Hickey EM. Diagnosis of dementia, clinical and pathophysiological signs of various etiologies. In: Dementia, from diagnosis to management - a functional approach. New York: Psychology Press; 2009. p. 9–39.
26. Ministry of Health, Labour and Welfare. The present status of the elderly with dementia, 2010. (in Japanese). 2013. http://www.mhlw.go.jp/stf/houdou_kouhou/kaiken_shiryou/2013/dl/130607-01.pdf. Accessed 15 Mar 2018.
27. Asada T, Taira M, Ishiai S, Kiyohara Y, Ikeda M, Suwa S, et al. Prevalence of dementia in the urban area and coping with life functioning disorders. In: Asada T (eds) A Report on Comprehensive research project for dementia countermeasures. (in Japanese). http://mhlw-grants.niph.go.jp/niph/search/NIDD00.do?resrchNum=201218011A. Accessed 17 Mar 2018.
28. Shigeta M. Epidemiology: rapid increase in Alzheimer's disease prevalence in Japan. Psychogeriatrics. 2004;4:117–9.

29. Luepker RV, Lakshminarayan K. Cardiovascular and cerebrovascular diseases. In: Detels R, Beaglehole R, Langsang MA, Gulliford M, editors. Oxford textbook of public health. 5th ed. Oxford: Oxford University Press; 2009. p. 971–96.
30. Ninomiya T, Ohara T, Hirakawa Y, Yoshida D, Doi Y, Hata J, et al. Midlife and late-life blood pressure and dementia in Japanese elderly: the hisayama study. Hypertension. 2011;58(1):22–8.
31. Fratiglioni L, Paillard-Borg S, Winblad B. An active and socially integrated lifestyle in late life might protect against dementia. Lancet Neurol. 2004;3(6):343–53.
32. Tanaka H, Iso H, Yokoyama T, Yoshiike N, Kokubo Y. Cerebrovascular disease. In: Detels R, McEwen J, Beaglehole R, Tanaka H, editors. Oxford textbook of public health. 4th ed. Oxford: Oxford University Press; 2004. p. 1193–226.
33. Wakabayashi K. The recent falling birthrate and the aging population issue in East Asia. Aziya Kenkyu (Asian Stud). 2006;52(2):95–112. (in Japanese)
34. Wu Y. The care of the elderly in Japan. New York: RoutledgeCurzon; 2004.
35. Sowers KM, Rowe WS. Global aging. In: Blackburn JA, Dulmus CN, editors. Handbook of gerontology, evidence-based approaches to theory, practice, and policy. Hoboken: John Willey & Sons, Inc.; 2007. p. 3–16.
36. Tu H, Wen CP, Tsai SP, Chow WH, Wen C, Ye Y, et al. Cancer risk associated with chronic diseases and disease markers: prospective cohort study. BMJ. 2018;36:k134. https://doi.org/10.1136/bmj.k134.
37. Ueno C. Sociology of the care, way to the welfare society of the person concerned sovereignty. Tokyo: Ohta Shuppan; 2011. (in Japanese)
38. Decker K, Maruyama A. Review of literature on father's recognition. Nihon Nouson Igakukai Zasshi (J Jpn Assoc Rural Med). 2015;64(4):718–24. (in Japanese)
39. Ministry of Education, Culture, Sports, Science and Technology, Japan. Improvement of higher education. In: A 2016 White Paper. (in Japanese). 2017. http://www.mext.go.jp/b_menu/hakusho/html/hpab201701/1389013.htm. Accessed 8 Mar 2018.
40. Chiba T. Life-style and sense of labor. In: Sato H, Sato A, editors. Sociology of work. Tokyo: Yuhikaku Publishing; 2007. p. 87–102. (in Japanese).
41. Kamibayashi C. Accepting foreign workers in Japanese Society, the Dilemma of a Temporary Immigrants Program. Tokyo: University of Tokyo Press; 2015. (in Japanese)

Chapter 2
Burden Among Family Caregivers of Older People Who Need Care in Japan

Masakazu Washio, Yasuko Toyoshima, Ikuko Miyabayashi, and Yumiko Arai

Abstract Improvements of public health and advances in medicine after World War II have given Japan one of the highest average life expectancies in the world. Increased life expectancy means that more senior citizens will have serious physical and mental illness, which causes an increase in the number of the older people who need care for their daily livings as well as medical care for their chronic diseases. Informal care for the older people with disabilities has proven to be a heavy burden for their family caregivers in many countries, and women were assumed to provide the main source of support for family members in Western countries as well as in Japan. The value of filial piety, which is a social norm that parents should love and care for their children and that children in turn should respect and care for their parents, have been shared for many generations in East Asian nations including Japan. Therefore, Japanese caregivers are concerned about what others say when they use social care services for their parents. In April 2000, the public long-term care insurance system (LTCIS) for the older people was launched in Japan, making it the third country, after the Netherlands and Germany. In this chapter, we would like to introduce Japanese LTCIS and studies on burden/depression among caregivers before and after the introduction of this system.

Keywords Older people · Family caregiver · Burden · Depression · Long-term care

M. Washio (✉)
Department of Community Health and Clinical Epidemiology, St. Mary's College, Kurume City, Fukuoka, Japan
e-mail: washiomasa@yahoo.co.jp

Y. Toyoshima
Yokkaichi Nursing and Medical Care University, Yokkaichi City, Mie, Japan

I. Miyabayashi
School of Nursing, Fukuoka University, Fukuoka City, Fukuoka, Japan

Y. Arai
Department of Gerontological Policy, National Center for Geriatrics and Gerontology (NCGG), Morioka-cho, Obu City, Aichi, Japan

2.1   Introduction

Before World War II, the average life expectancy was shorter than 50 years (i.e., 43 years old for men and 44 years old for women in the 1890s and 46.9 years old for men and 49.6 years old for women in 1935) in Japan [1]. However, improvement of public health and advances in medicine after World War II have given Japan one of the highest average life expectancies in the world (i.e., 81.0 years old for men and 87.1 years old for women in 2016) [2], and the proportion of the elderly (i.e., 65 years old and older) increased from 4.9% in 1950 to 26.6% in 2015 [2]. The dramatic increase in the number of older people in this country is well documented [3]. Increased life expectancy means that more senior citizens will have serious physical and mental illness, which causes an increase in the number of senior citizens who need care in their daily lives. It is estimated that the number of older people with disabilities will reach 5.2 million in 2020 [4]. Demand for long-term care grows exponentially with age, and the bulk is much greater in the older ages (aged 75 years and older) than younger ages (younger than 75 years old) among the elderly.

In former days, family members took care of the disabled elderly with chronic illness in the traditional family system because most Japanese elderly, over 60% compared with 20% or less in Western countries, lived with their children [3].

For most adult children who live with the their parents before their parents develop chronic illnesses such as dementia, the change in role identity is a slow process, and the care needs of the aged parents may gradually increase, which may lead adult children to undertaking a family-caregiver identity without experiencing heavy stress [5]. Women were assumed to provide the main source of support for family members in Western countries [6] as well as in Japan [7, 8]. The value of filial piety, which is a social norm where parents should love and care for their children and that the children in turn should respect and care for their parents, have been shared for many generations in East Asian nations (China, Korea, and Japan) [9]. The study by Lee and Farran [10] compared depressive symptoms among South Korean, Korean-American, and Caucasian-American female family caregivers of older persons with dementia. In their study, the rates of the daughter and daughter-in-law (i.e., son's wife) were greater than the rates of the wife in South Korean caregivers (81.0% vs. 16.0%) and in Korean-American caregivers (71.2% vs. 23.7%), while the rates of two groups were almost similar in Caucasian-American caregivers (50.0% vs. 48.7%) [10].

In contrast to Nordic countries where the ultimate responsibilities lies with the state rather than the family iteself, in Japan, the family care was the gratuious labor that a married woman performs among families [7, 8] and female family members (i.e., daughters, daughters-in-law (i.e., son's wives), and wives) took care of aged family members under the influence of Confucianism (i.e., filial piety) [8]. However, the number of children in each family has dramatically decreased because the live birth rate (per every 1000 Japanese people) decreased from 28.1 in 1950 to 7.8 in 2016 [2]. According to the decreased birth rate, the average number of family members in each family decreased from 3.41 in 1970 to 2.42 in 2010 [11], which decreased power of family caregiving. Furthermore, the proportion of full-time workers increased from 31.8% in 1985 to 41.9% in 2010 among Japanese women with working age (i.e., 15–64 years old), while the proportion of those who take care of the housework for their family decreased from 34.8% in 1985 to 26.3% in 2010 [11], which also decreased the ability of family caregiving. In addition, the proportion of the elderly who lived with their children decreased from 69.0% in 1980 to 39.0% in 2015 [12], while the proportion of those who lived with their spouses only increased from 19.6% in 1980 to 38.9% in 2015 [12], which increased the rate of spouse-caregivers and male-caregivers among family caregivers of older people with disabilities in Japan.

Nowadays, many Japanese family caregivers often have to take care of their charges without help from other relatives, because they often live too far away to provide assistance from their relatives. Therefore, family caregivers are often both physically and mentally burdened with caring for their charges [4]. Except spouse-caregivers (i.e., retired husbands and wives, full-time homemakers), other family caregivers (i.e., daughters, sons, son's wives) may be obliged to change their work from full-time to part-time or to retire before a retirement age in order to take care of the charges at home in Japan [7], which may financially burden caregivers as well.

Several reports [13, 14] demonstrated that a large amount of time spent on daily caregiving was related to the feeling among such caregivers of carrying an insupportable burden. It has been reported that caring for older people may induce depression in the caregivers [15]. Caregiver's depression is an important social problem in Japan because it involves the potential risk of caregivers discontinuing caregiving at home [16].

2.2 Public Long-Term Care Insurance System for Older People in Japan

Long-term care services are needed for persons with long-standing physical or mental disabilities, who need assistance with basic activities of daily living (ADL) (e.g., bathing, dressing, eating, getting in and out of bed or chairs, moving around, and using the bathroom), many of whom are the highest age groups of the population (i.e., older people aged over 80) [17].

In Japan, the environment for older people and their caregivers has undergone momentous changes. In April 2000, to promote greater autonomy of the older people in their daily lives as well as to reduce burden on their caregivers, the public long-term care insurance system (LTCIS) for older people was launched in Japan, making it the third country [18, 19], after the Netherlands [20] and Germany [21], to provide such insurance.

The fundamental purpose of LTCIS is the establishment of what can be called "universalism" in care policies for older people [22]. First, under the new public

LTCIS, all of the older people in Japan, who need assistance with basic ADL, can use the care services for the older people, according to the Government-Certified Disability Index (GCDI) (i.e., degree of need of care; "Yokaigodo" in Japanese) [23], while the care services for the older people in Japan were formerly reserved for users from low-income households before LTCIS was implemented (i.e., under the old selective tax scheme). Second, the users themselves can determine their individual need for services under LTCIS, while the administration of service was determined by public administrative agencies before LTCIS [19]. Under LTCIS, the older people and their caregivers are entitled to decide both the kind and the amount of services they wish to use according to their need of care within the limits of GCDI [19, 23] (i.e., degree of need of care). Third, LTCIS allows both profit-based and nonprofit private organizations to provide care services for older people, while the service providers were confined to municipal governments and nonprofit private organizations stipulated by the Social Welfare Law before LTCIS. Fourth, the insured persons are required to bear the co-payment (i.e., 10%) depending on the service utilized under LTCIS, while the older people (65.0 years old and older) paid only limited fees before LTCIS. Last, the middle aged (40–64 years old) are also required to become members of LTCIS in order to assist in bearing the cost of this insurance system, due to their parents possibly using services under LTCIS.

However, some problems about the LTCIS were pointed out before its introduction [24]. First, the insurer is not a country but cities, towns, and villages which have big variability in financial power. Therefore, the quality and the kind of care services that insured persons receive as well as share of insurance premiums may be different between insurers (i.e., cities, towns, and villages) [24]. Second, family care is still the gratuitous labor even after the introduction of the LTCIS in Japan. In contrast, German family caregivers receive money of reward for caring for older people at home, although they receive much less money than "performance in kind" to provide public assistance by furnishing care services [24], which suppress the expenditure and may evade large deficits in Germany.

After Japan, South Korea launched a public long-term care insurance system (LTCIS) for older people in 2008 [25]. Ham [25] pointed out several problems about the LTCIS in South Korea such as (1) deficiencies in the system and service contents, (2) problems with privatization of care services (e.g., commercial operation, lower service levels, workers' wage exploitation, and worsening worker conditions), (3) difficult accessibility to service use, (4) regional disparity in services, and (5) improper self-paid insurance premiums (i.e., decreased usage of services in the poor senior citizens and increased usage of services in rich senior citizens).

In Japan, under LTCIS, the insured senior citizens (65.0 years old and older) increased from 21.65 million in 2000 to 33.87 million in 2016, while the senior citizens in need of care increased from 2.18 million in 2000 to 6.22 million in 2016 [2]. The older people with disabilities can use services according to their GCDI (i.e., degree of need of care) under LTCIS. However, some of the senior citizens are obliged to abandon their right to use certain parts of the services under LTCIS due to not being able to afford the self-pay financial burden of all the services that they have the right to use according to their GCDI. Before the introduction of LTCIS, the senior citizens in the poor class did not have to pay money to use any service under the old selective tax scheme. On the other hand, after the introduction of LTCIS, only the very poor senior citizens who live on welfare do not have to pay money (i.e., the co-payment) for care services under LTCIS. Therefore, the poor senior citizens, those who do not live on welfare, have more difficulty accessing the care services under LTCIS than under the old selective tax scheme. On the other hand, with reduced self-payment under LTCIS and the ability to use care services with the co-payment (10%), the senior citizens in the middle and upper class can use more services under LTCIS than under the old selective tax scheme. After saving 90% of money for care services under LTCIS, they can pay for more additional services out of pocket.

After the revision of LTCIS, the financial support to reduce the financial burden of the poor senior citizens was offered, while the rate of co-payment was increased from 10% to 20% for the rich senior citizens (i.e., one fifth of the older people) in 2015 [2]. However, ownership of expensive real estate does not always mean that the senior citizens and their caregivers are rich enough to pay higher rate (20%) of self-payment for care services under LTCIS. Although some of the frail elderly and their caregivers (e.g., the older people with disabilities and their spouses aged over 80 years old, the older people with disabilities and their adult children who have no income) live in the residents at the place with high land prices, these older people with disabilities and family caregivers may abandon their right to use parts of the services under LTCIS, because they do not have enough money (i.e., income or savings in their banks) to pay higher rates (20%) of self-payment for all care services that they have the right to use according to their GCDI (i.e., degree of need of care).

In Nordic countries such as Sweden, the ultimate responsibility for the older people with disabilities lies with the state rather than with the family itself [26]. Mikami [26] reported the five basic ideas of welfare for the older people in Sweden, which were normalization (i.e., continue to live in the usual living environment), view a person as a whole (i.e., view a person from psychological, physical, and social aspects), self-determination (i.e., recognize and respect rights to decide one's way of life), social participation (i.e., take part in community activities), and activation (i.e., assist the elderly to perform leisure activities according to his/her ability and interests).

Maintaining an active life is believed to help the older people to preserve their physical and mental health [27]. Fratiglioni et al. [27] suggested that all of the social, mental, and physical lifestyle components have a protective effect against dementia. Therefore, the older people should not change their residence in late life. However, there are a few older people who sell their residence in order to use care services under LTCIS. For the prevention of dementia, the care system for the older people to cover the minimum care services for all older people with no co-payment may be desirable in order to ensure the safety net for the older people.

2.3 Burden Among Family Caregivers of Older People

2.3.1 *Factors Related to a Heavy Burden/Depression Among Family Caregivers of Older Persons with Disabilities*

Informal care for the older persons with disabilities has proved to be a heavy burden and source of depression for family caregivers [28–35].

Table 2.1 illustrates the factors related to the burden/depression among family caregivers of the older persons with disabilities in Japan.

2.3.1.1 The Characteristics of the Older Persons Who Are Cared by Their Family Caregivers

Older persons with severe dementia [33, 35], older persons who have behavioral and psychological symptoms of dementia (BPSD) [32–34, 36], and older persons of the male sex [34–39] show a positive association with an increased risk of burden among family caregivers, while older persons with severe limitations in activities of daily living (ADL) (i.e., bedridden elderly) are less likely to increase the risk of a heavy burden than older persons with light/moderate limited ADL [32]. These findings may be partly explained in the following ways. First, most caregivers are females (e.g., wives, daughters, son's wives) in Japan. Second, it may be more physically burdensome to care for males than females because males are heavier than females.

Table 2.1 Factors related to heavy burden/depression among family caregivers of older people with disabilities in Japan

Factors	Association	References
(1) Characteristics of older people with disabilities		
Severe dementia	Positive	[33, 35]
Behavioral and psychological symptoms of dementia	Positive	[32–34, 36]
Male sex	Positive	[34–39]
Severe limitation of ADL (persons with dementia)	Inverse	[32]
(2) Characteristics of the family caregivers		
Spouses	Positive	[34, 37, 38]
Aged caregivers	Positive	[35–37]
Be in ill health	Positive	[35, 38, 39]
With chronic diseases	Positive	[34, 37, 38, 40]
Be concern about what others say	Positive	[37, 40]
With an adequate income	Inverse	[35]
(3) Care setting		
Daily caregiving time	Positive	[33–38]
Have no hour relieved of their duties	Positive	[33, 34, 38]
Find it convenient to use services	Inverse	[33]

Second, it may be more difficult to care for male patients with dementia than female patients with dementia when patients have behavioral problems because males are generally physically stronger than females. Third, patients with severe dementia may have many BPSD. Last, older persons with dementia, who have severe limitations of ADL (i.e., bedridden elderly), are not able either to leave their bed in order to use violence on their caregivers or to wander around, while the older persons with dementia, who have light/moderate limitation of ADL, are able to do so.

2.3.1.2 The Characteristics of Family Caregivers

Spouse-caregivers [34, 37, 38], aged caregivers [35–37], those with ill health [35, 38, 39], those with chronic diseases [34, 37, 38, 40], and caregivers who are concerned about what others say [37, 40] are more likely to feel a heavier burden than their counterparts, while caregivers who have an adequate income [35] are less likely to feel a heavy burden than their counterparts.

The proportion of the senior citizens (i.e., 65 years old and older) was 27.3% in 2016 [2]. Among the households with senior citizens, 31.1% are households of only a married couple (husband and wife) [2]. Husbands and wives care for their disabled spouses with obligation and love in Japan [7]. However, old spouse-caregivers with chronic diseases may have uneasiness toward health. They may be afraid that there is nobody who will take care of their husbands/wives if they themselves are greatly impacted by their own disease.

Caregivers who are concerned about what others say [37, 40] are more likely to feel a heavier burden than their counterparts. Arai et al. [41, 42] reported that caregivers of the disabled elderly who are concerned about what others think or say were less likely to use public services than those who did not. Those who are concerned about what others say may feel a heavy burden because they hesitate to use social services under LTCIS.

2.3.1.3 The Care Setting

Caregivers who spend a long time with daily caregiving [33–38] and those who cannot go out without their charges/ those who have no hours relieved of their duties [33, 34, 38] are more likely to feel a heavier burden than their counterparts, while caregivers who find it convenient to use services [33] are less likely to do so than their counterparts. A heavy burden among caregivers may increase the risk of discontinuation of caregiving [16, 43] or inadequate care (i.e., abuse) [44, 45]. Therefore, we should provide enough social services for the frail elderly and their family caregivers in order to reduce time spent on daily caregiving and to give caregivers hours free from caregiving. Furthermore, caregiver's concern about what others say deters caregivers from using social services [41, 42]. Education not only for the frail elderly and their caregivers but also for the general population is needed so that anyone can use social services without feeling humiliated.

2.3.2 Factors Related to Ill Health Among Family Caregivers of Older Persons in Japan

Family caregivers are often both physically and mentally burdened with caring for older persons at home [4, 46].

A cross-sectional study was conducted in order to evaluate the factors related to ill health among 344 family caregivers of the older persons with home-visiting nursing services [47]. In this study, a Japanese version of the Center for Epidemiologic Studies Depression (CES-D) scale [48, 49] and a Japanese version of the Zarit Caregiver Burden Interview (J-ZBI) [50–52] were used to evaluate the depressive state and burden of family caregivers. Among them, 134 caregivers (39.0%) answered that they were in ill health, while 210 caregivers (61.0%) answered that they were in good health [47]. Caregivers in ill health were older (66.2 ± 12.2 years old vs. 60.6 ± 13.5 years old, $p < 0.05$) and more depressed (CES-D, 20.5 ± 10.4 vs. 13.5 ± 9.0, $p < 0.05$) and felt a heavier burden (J-ZBI, 13.5 ± 9.0 vs. 29.2 ± 17.5, $p < 0.05$) than those in good health [41]. Compared with their counterparts, they were more likely to be spousal caregivers (57.5% vs. 37.1%, $p < 0.05$) and less likely to be adult children caregivers (25.4% vs. 25.4%, $p < 0.05$) and were more likely to care for males (52.2% vs. 35.7%, $p < 0.05$) than those in good health [47]. In addition, family caregivers with ill health are more likely to take care of older persons who have behavioral and psychological symptoms of dementia than their counterparts (33.6% vs. 20.5%, $p < 0.05$) [47]. Furthermore, home-help service (61.9% vs. 46.2%, $p < 0.05$) was more commonly used in caregivers in ill health than those in good health. Even after controlling for other factors, depression (odds ratio = 2.04, 95% confidence interval: 1.18–3.57), spousal caregivers (odds ratio = 1.92, 95% confidence interval: 1.19–3.13), caring for older persons who have behavioral and psychological symptoms of dementia (odds ratio = 1.96, 95% confidence interval: 1.14–3.33), and the usage of home-help services (odds ratio = 1.67, 95% confidence interval: 1.03–2.70) were associated with an increased risk of ill health among family caregivers [47]. Since this study was a cross-sectional study, the usage of a home-help service may not be the cause of ill health but the result of ill health among family caregivers. The finding in this study is consistent with the result of the study in Australia [53], which showed an inverse association between well-being and burden as well as a positive association between depression and burden among caregivers of persons with dementia.

Among the community-dwelling Japanese senior citizens (i.e., 65 years old and older), 68.2% of males and 69.1% of female had chronic diseases and attended hospitals as outpatients in 2016, while, among the community-dwelling Japanese advanced elderly persons (i.e., 75 years old and older), 72.5% of males and 73.0% of females did so in 2016 [2]. On the other hand, among the community-dwelling Japanese in their 50s (i.e., 50–59 years old), 41.2% of males and 42.6% of females had chronic diseases and attended hospitals as outpatients in 2016 [2]. Therefore, it may be plausible that older caregivers such as spouse-caregivers are more likely to feel ill health than younger caregivers such as adult child caregivers.

2.3.3 Depressive Rates Among Family Caregivers of the Older People Around the Introduction of Public Long-Term Care Insurance System for the Older People in Japan

The rates of depressed family caregivers of the senior citizens who used home-visiting nursing services around the time of the introduction of the public long-term care insurance system (LTCIS) for the older people were 50.3–56.3% [34, 54] before LTCIS and 34.2–48.4% [34, 35, 54] after LTCIS. The rate of depression among caregivers only slightly decreased after LTCIS compared with the rate before LTCIS. However, the rate of depression is much higher than the rate of depression among the community-dwelling older people (5.3%) [49]. Since a caregiver's depression is a risk factor for the discontinuation of caregiving [16], care managers and municipal public nurses should take care of not only the older persons with disabilities but also caregivers in order to prevent caregivers' depression.

Before LTCIS, caregivers who consulted with physicians about their own health (odds ratio = 2.99, 95% confidence interval: 1.60–5.60), those who felt ill health (odds ratio = 5.17, 95% confidence interval: 2.71–9.87), those who cared for older persons who have behavioral and psychological symptoms of dementia (odds ratio = 2.75, 95% confidence interval: 1.44–5.25), and those who attended the elderly more than 16 h/day (odds ratio = 2.77, 95% confidence interval: 1.36–5.67) showed a positive association with the depression of caregivers after controlling for caregiver's age and sex, district, and life events (e.g., death of family members, divorce, loss of employment) [34]. On the other hand, after LTCIS, caregivers who were spouses (odds ratio = 2.92, 95% confidence interval: 1.42–6.01), those who consulted with physicians about their own health (odds ratio = 4.01, 95% confidence interval: 1.97–8.17), those who felt ill health (odds ratio = 6.19, 95% confidence interval: 2.92–13.12), those who cared for males (odds ratio = 2.79, 95% confidence interval: 1.35–5.74), those who cared for older persons who have behavioral and psychological symptoms of dementia (odds ratio = 2.35, 95% confidence interval: 1.14–4.81), and those who could not go out without accompanying their charges (odds ratio = 2.78, 95% confidence interval: 1.30–5.88) were associated with an increased risk of depression after controlling for caregiver's age and sex, district, and life events [34].

2.3.4 The Characteristics of the Home-Visiting Nursing Service Users Under the Public Long-Term Care Insurance System

As shown in Table 2.2, home-visiting nursing service users increased from 198,839 in September 2007 to 265,024 in September 2013 [55, 56], which means that the number of home-visiting nursing service users increased by 30% during this

Table 2.2 The number of home-visiting nursing service users and the number and proportion of users utilizing medical care

Medical care by home-visiting nurses	September 2007 $n = 198839$	September 2013 $n = 265024$
Medication administration and management	95364 (48.0%)	137784 (52.0%)
Management for patients who need enema and stool extraction	51844 (26.1%)	62882 (23.7%)
Management for patients with decubitus ulcer	75809 (38.1%)	82427 (31.1%)
Support for patients with home oxygen therapy	16368 (8.2%)	22294 (8.4%)
Management for patients with tracheotomy cannula	6837 (3.4%)	8831 (3.3%)
Management for patients with mechanical ventilation	4605 (2.3%)	8264 (3.1%)
Management for patients with gastric fistula catheter	22648 (11.4%)	22520 (9.6%)
Management of patients with tube feeding	10716 (5.4%)	6069 (2.3%)
Management for patients with intravenous hyperalimentation	1880 (0.9%)	3470(1.3%)
Management for patients with bladder dwelling balloon catheter	22526 (11.3%)	28469 (10.7%)
Management for patients undergoing chemotherapy for cancer	670 (0.3%)	1380 (0.5%)
Management for patients who need pain control with medicine	5088 (2.6%)	5088 (2.6%)

This table is made from the data of "National Survey of Nursing-Care Service Facilities" in e-Stat (Portal Site of Official Statistics of Japan) (https://www.e-stat.go.jp) [56]

period. Among them, almost 50% of the users needed "medication administration and management" by home-visiting nurses, over 30% of users received medical care for their decubitus ulcer, over 10% of users needed care for their bladder dwelling balloon catheter, almost 10% of users had gastric fistula catheters, and over 8% of users needed support for home oxygen therapy. Although the proportion was small, home-visiting nurses took care of the patients with mechanical ventilation, those with intravenous hyperalimentation, and those with chemotherapy for cancer as well.

However, all users cannot use home-visiting nursing services every day. Under LTCIS, the frail elderly have to use the care services for the older peoples according to the Government-Certified Disability Index (GCDI) (i.e., degree of need of care), which means that older persons themselves have to pay 100% of the charge for the usage of services greater than the limits under LTCIS. Therefore, all users cannot use home-visiting nursing services every day, and not a few family caregivers may feel caregiver's burden because caregivers themselves have to take care of the older persons who need medical care at home after nurses return to the nursing stations.

2.3.5 Caring for Cancer Patients at Home

Cancer is a leading cause of death for the general population as well as for senior citizens in Japan [2]. Cancer patients are often not discharged from hospitals because of severe pain, and pain management is one of the most important factors for the cancer patients to stay at home. Although the proportion was small, home-visiting nurses took care of cancer patients undergoing chemotherapy (0.3–0.5%) as well as cancer patients who need pain control with the medicine (2.6%) [55, 56]. Hashimoto et al. [57] reported that more than half (56%) of cancer patients with home palliative care had severe pain. There may be different responses to the pain medicine between the patients. In their survey, 259 out of 290 cancer patients lived with family [57]. As problems in family care, 116 family members (40%) felt a burden of caregiving, while 41 patients (14%) had no family caregivers. Among 284 patients who were followed until death, 242 patients (85%) died at home [57]. Among these patients who died at home, 238 patients (98%) used home-visiting nursing service, and 127 patients (52%) received strong opioids [57].

Ishi et al. [58] reported that family caregivers who cared for terminal cancer patients at home experienced several difficulties. Cancer patients showed excruciating pain even with pain medicine and difficulty in caring due to the reluctance of using opioids [58]. When there is a difference in opinions between family members as to pain control due to side effects such as sedation by opioids, caregivers may feel difficulties in utilizing nursing interventions. Due to these problems, family caregivers agonized about facing the limitations of caregiving due to increasing pain in the patients [58], which may increase the burden of family caregivers. Some caregivers were modest and hesitated to ask a nurse to come and care for cancer patients at night, while others thought that home-visiting nurses were not trained well enough to care for cancer patients at home [58]. These findings suggest that well-trained home-visiting nurses may play an important role in caring for patients with medical care such as cancer patients at home.

2.4 Discussion

Improvement of public health and advances in medicine after World War II have given Japan one of the highest life expectancies in the world (i.e., 81.0 years for males and 87.1 years for females in 2016) [2]. The number of older people is estimated to increase from 33.9 million in 2015 to 37.8 million in 2035 [2]. On the other hand, live birth rate (per 1000 Japanese population) decreased from 28.1 in 1950 [59] to 7.8 in 2016 [2]. Because the birth rate dropped sharply after the postwar baby boom, population aging is proceeding more rapidly than any other industrialized nation [3]. The increased number of older people led to an increase in the

Table 2.3 The proportion of males and females who have chronic diseases and attend hospitals as outpatients among Japanese in the community

Year of national survey	1998 [59] (%)	2001 [60] (%)	2007 [61] (%)	2016 [2] (%)
Males (general population)	25.9	28.7	31.1	37.2
Males aged 65 years old and over	59.9	60.9	62.9	68.2
Males aged 75 years old and over	63.1	64.3	67.6	72.5
Females (general population)	30.8	33.9	35.5	40.7
Females aged 65 years old and over	64.5	64.8	64.5	69.1
Females aged 75 years old and over	66.9	66.9	67.5	73.0

Comprehensive survey of living conditions, list of statistical surveys conducted by Ministry of Health, Labour and Welfare (www.mhlw.go.jp)

Health and Welfare Statistics Association (2000). Trend of national health 2000. Tokyo: Health and Welfare Statistics Association (in Japanese)

Health and Welfare Statistics Association (2004). Trend of national health 2004. Tokyo: Health and Welfare Statistics Association (in Japanese)

Health and Welfare Statistics Association (2010). Trend of national health 2010–2011. Tokyo: Health and Welfare Statistics Association (in Japanese)

Health, Labour and Welfare Statistics Association (2017). Trend of national health 2017–2018. Tokyo: Health, Labour and Welfare Statistics Association (in Japanese)

number of the older persons with chronic diseases. As shown in Table 2.3, the proportion of those who have chronic diseases and attend hospitals as outpatients increased from 56.9% for males and 64.5% for females in 1998 [58] to 68.2% for males and 69.1% for females in 2016 [2] among the older people who live in the community in Japan. These findings may suggest that the older people who need medical care increased in the community during these 20 years and will increase from now on for a while.

In 1972, the free medical care programs for the older people started at the national level, and the regular health insurance system raised the coverage ratio to 100% for the older patients, paid for by the Finance Ministry subsidy [3]. Today, however, consumers (the older persons with disabilities) have to pay a 10% nursing service/caring service fee under LTCIS because the coverage ratio is 90% for users [2]. Since financial burden was found to be related to a heavier burden of family caregivers [35], a financial burden may restrain caregivers from using social services. Care managers and municipal public nurses should help family caregivers so that they can use free services such as municipal services and informal services.

Washio et al. [47] found that depression increased the risk of ill health among family caregivers even after controlling for other factors. On the other hand, Oura et al. [34] reported that caregivers who consulted with physicians about their own health had an increased risk of depression, even after controlling for other factors. Since caregiver's depression increases the risk of the discontinuation of caregiving [16], it may be one of the most important requirements for successful caregiving that the aged caregivers take care of caregivers themselves as well as their aged charges especially when old caregivers care for older persons with disabilities. In order to reduce caregiver's burden as well as to prevent caregivers' ill health, municipal public nurses should help family caregivers feel free to use municipal services for the older persons with disabilities.

Spending a long time caring for an older person with disabilities every day is suggested to increase the burden of family caregivers [33–38], while having time relieved of their duties is suggested to reduce the burden of family caregivers [33, 34, 38]. In order to reduce caregiver's burden, care managers should advise family caregivers to use respite care services, which give caregivers a short-term break from their usual care commitment. Informal care provided by other family members, relatives, friends, or neighbors is also helpful to give family caregivers a short time break from their duties as well as to reduce the sense of loneliness among family caregivers, which may also reduce the burden of family caregivers.

In conclusion, in order to promote greater autonomy of the older persons with disabilities as well as to reduce the burden on their family caregivers, LTCIS was launched in Japan. In our studies [34, 35, 54], however, the proportion of depressed family caregivers were 50.3–56.3% before LTCIS and 34.2–48.4% after LTCIS. These findings may suggest that the rate of depressed family caregivers only slightly decreased after LTCIS compared with the rate prior to LTCIS. In Japan, there may be several barriers for the older people and their caregivers to access social services. Some caregivers may hesitate to use social services because they are concerned about what others say under the influence of Confucianism (i.e., children should care for their parents by themselves), while others may abandon their right to use a part of services under LTCIS because they do not have enough money for the co-payment for all care services that they have the right to use under LTCIS. We should remove the barriers for older persons with disabilities and their caregivers to use social services under the LTCIS. Education for the community residents should be recommended so that anyone can use social services without feeling humiliated. In addition, municipal services and/or informal services should be provided when the older people and their caregivers cannot afford to use social service under the LTCIS.

References

1. Ministry of Health and Welfare. Annual report of health and welfare. Tokyo: Ministry of Health and Welfare; 1978. (In Japanese). http://www.mhlw.go.jp/toukei_hakusho/hakusho/kousei/1978/dl/03.pdf. Accessed 19 Dec 2017
2. Health, Labour and Welfare Statistics Association. Trend of national health 2017–2018. Tokyo: Health, Labour and Welfare Statistics Association; 2017. (in Japanese)
3. Cambell JC. How policies change: the Japanese government and the aging society. Princeton: Princeton University Press; 1992.
4. Maeda D. The outline of new public long-term care insurance program. In: Takagi F, editor. Aging in Japan, vol. 2003. Tokyo: Japan Aging Research Center; 2003. p. 188–91.
5. Montogomery RJV, Rowe JM, Kosloski K. Family caregiving. In: Blackburn JA, Dulmus CN, editors. Handbook of gerontology: evidence-based approaches to theory, practice, and policy. Hoboken, NJ: John Willey & Sons, Inc.; 2007. p. 426–54.

6. Barnes M. Caring and social justice. New York: Palgrave Macmillan; 2006.
7. Ueno C. Sociology of the care, way to the welfare society of the person concerned sovereignty. Tokyo: Ohta Shuppan; 2011. (in Japanese)
8. Arai Y, Ikegami N. How will Japan cope with the impending surge of dementia? In: Wimo A, Jönsson B, Karlson G, Winblad A, editors. Health economics of dementia. Chichester: John Wiley & Sons; 1998. p. 275–84.
9. Sung KT (2007). Respect and care for the elderly: the East Asian way, Lanham, MD: University Press of America Inc.
10. Lee EE, Farran CJ. Depression among Korean, Korean American, and Caucasian American family caregivers. J Transcult Nurs. 2004;15(1):18–25.
11. Statistics Bureau, Ministry of Internal Affairs and Communications. 2010 national census: the Japanese population and household according to the life-stage. Tokyo: Ministry of Internal Affairs and Communications; 2014. (in Japanese). http://www.stat.go.jp/data/kokusei/2010/life.htm. Accessed 19 Dec 2017
12. Cabinet Office, Government of Japan. Koureishakai Hakusho 2017 (White paper for the Aged Society 2017). Tokyo: Cabinet Office, Government of Japan; 2017. (in Japanese)
13. Rabins PV, Fitting MD, Esatham J, et al. Emotional adaptation over time in caregivers for chronically ill elderly people. Age Aging. 1990;19:185–90.
14. Walker AJ, Acock AC, Bowman SR, et al. Amount of care given and caregiving satisfaction: a latent growth curve analysis. J Gerontol B Psychol Sci Soc Sci. 1996;51(B):130–42.
15. Barnes CL, Given BA, Given CW. Caregivers of elderly relatives; spouses and adult children. Health Soc Work. 1992;17:282–9.
16. Arai Y, Sugiura M, Washio M, Miura H, Kudo K. Caregiver depression predicts early discontinuation of care for disabled elderly at home. Psychiatry Clin Neurosci. 2001;55:379–82.
17. Organisation for Economic Co-operation and Development. The OECD health project, long-term care for older people. Paris: OECD Publishing; 2005. ISBN 92-64-00848-9
18. Arai Y. Insurance for long-term care planned in Japan. Lancet. 1997;350:1831.
19. Arai Y, Kudo K, Washio M. Caring for Japan's elderly. Lancet. 1998;352:1393.
20. Campen C, Gameren E. Eligibility for long-term care in the Netherlands: development of a decision support system. Health Soc Care Community. 2005;13:287–96.
21. Tesch-Romer C. Intergenerational solidarity and caregiving. Z Gerontol Geriatr. 2001;34:28–33.
22. Shimizu Y. Development of public long term care insurance and future direction of the elderly care. In: Takagi F, editor. Aging in Japan, vol. 2003. Tokyo: Japan Aging Research Center; 2003. p. 197–204.
23. Arai Y, Zarit SH, Kumamoto K, Takeda A. Are there inequities in the assessment of dementia under Japan's LTC insurance system? Int J Geriatr Psychiatry. 2003;18:346–52.
24. Yamada M. Characteristic of the care service and policy: comparison between Japan and Germany. In: Nishimura S, editor. Iryohakusho (Annual report of medical care). Tokyo: Nihon-iryo-kikaku; 1998. p. 45–73. (in Japanese).
25. Ham IW. Long-term care insurance system of South Korea: achievements and issues at the point of one year from enforcement. Hyoron Shakaikagaku (Soc Sci Rev). 2010;90:75–97. (in Japanese)
26. Mikami F. Welfare services for the elderly. In: Maruo N, Shionoya Y, editors. Social security system of the advanced countries, social security in Sweden. Tokyo: University of Tokyo Press; 1999. p. 253–74. (in Japanese).
27. Fratiglioni L, Paillard-Borg S, Winblad B. An active and socially integrated lifestyle in late life might protect against dementia. Lancet Neurol. 2004;3:343–53.
28. Zarit SH, Reever KE, Bach-Peterson J. Relatives of the impaired elderly: Correlates of feelings of burden. Gerontologist. 1980;20:649–55.
29. Montgomery RJV, Gonyea JG, Hooyman NR. Caregiving and experience of subjective and objective burden. Fam Relat. 1985;34:19–26.
30. Fitting M, Rabins P, Lucas MJ, Eastham J. Caregivers for dementia patients: a comparison of husband and wives. Gerontologist. 1986;26:248–52.

31. Gallagher D, Rose J, Rivera P, Lovett S, Thompson LW. Prevalence of depression in family caregivers. Gerontologist. 1989;29:449–56.
32. Arai Y, Washio M. Burden felt by family caring for the elderly members needing care in southern Japan. Aging Ment Health. 1999;3:158–64.
33. Arai Y, Kumamoto K, Washio M, Ueda T, Miura H, Kudo K. Factors related to feelings of burden among caregivers looking after impaired elderly in Japan under the Long-Term Care Insurance System. Psychiatry Clin Neurosci. 2004;58:396–402.
34. Oura A, Washio M, Arai Y, Ide S, Yamasaki R, Wada J, Kuwahara Y, Mori M. Depression among caregivers of the frail elderly in Japan before and after the introduction of the public long-term care insurance system. Z Gerontol Geriatr. 2007;40:112–8.
35. Arai Y, Kumamoto K, Mizuno Y, Washio M. Depression among family caregivers of community-dwelling older people who used services under the long term care insurance program: a large-scale population-based study in Japan. Aging Ment Health. 2014;18(1): 81–91.
36. Washio M, Nogami Y, Motoyama S, Yamasaki R, Horiguchi I, Toyoshima Y. Burden among family caregivers of the elderly in need of care and factors related to their burden before and after the revision of public long-term care insurance system. Rinsho To Kenkyu. 2015;92(10):1311–6. (in Japanese)
37. Toyoshima Y, Washio M, Horiguchi I, Yamasaki R, Onimaru M, Nakamura K, Miyabayashi I, Arai Y. Undue concern for other's opinion is related to depression among family caregivers disabled elderly in southern Japan. Int Med J. 2016;23(1):30–3.
38. Washio M, Arai Y, Izumi H, Mori M. Burden on family caregivers of frail elderly persons one year after the introduction of public long term care insurance service in the Onga District, Fukuoka Prefecture: evaluation with a Japanese version of the Zarit caregiver burden interview. Nihon Ronen Igaku Zasshi. 2003;40:147–55. (in Japanese)
39. Washio M, Oura A, Arai Y, Mori M. Depression among caregivers of the frail elderly, three years after the introduction of public long-term care insurance for the elderly. Int Med J. 2003;10:179–83.
40. Washio M, Takeida K, Arai Y, Shang E, Oura A, Mori M. Depression among caregivers of the frail elderly with visiting nursing services in the northernmost city of Japan. Int Med J. 2015;22(4):250–3.
41. Arai Y, Sugiura M, Miura H, Washio M, Kudo K. Undue concern for other's opinions deters caregivers of impaired elderly from using public services in rural Japan. Int J Geriatr Psychiatry. 2000;15:961–8.
42. Arai Y, Washio M, Miura H, Kudo K. Dementia care in Japan: insurance for long term care legislation in Japan. Int J Geriatr Psychiatry. 1998;13:572–3.
43. Arai Y, Zarit SH, Sugiura M, Washio M. Patterns of outcome of caregiving for the impaired elderly: a longitudinal study in rural Japan. Aging Ment Health. 2002;6(1):39–46.
44. Ueda T. Inadequate care by family caregiver of frail elderly living at home. Nihon Koshu Eisei Zassgi. 2000;47(3):264–74. (in Japanese)
45. Nitta J, Kumamoto K, Arai Y. Burden felt by family caregivers of the elderly registered with visiting nurses' stations in Kyoto. Nihon Ronen Igaku Zasshi. 2005;42:181–5. (in Japanese)
46. Arai Y, Zarit SH. Exploring strategies to alleviate caregiver burden: effects of the national long-term care insurance scheme in Japan. Psychogeriatrics. 2011;11(3):183–9.
47. Washio M, Toyoshima Y, Arai Y. Factors related to ill health among family caregivers of the older people. 17th Annual Meeting of Japan Society of Health Promotion, Nisshin City, Aichi Prefecture, Japan, Feb 2016. (in Japanese).
48. Radloff L. The CES-D scale: a self-reported depression scale for research in the general population. Appl Psychol Meas. 1977;1:385–401.
49. Ihara K. Depressive states and their correlates in elderly people in a rural community. Nihon Koshu Eisei Zasshi. 1993;40(2):85–94. (in Japanese)
50. Zarit SH, Zarit JM. The memory and behavior problems checklist-1987R and the burden interview. Philadelphia, PA: Pennsylvania University; 1987.

51. Arai Y. The Japanese version of the Zarit Caregiver Burden Interview (J-ZBI). Nippon Rinsho. 2011;69(8):459–63. (in Japanese)
52. Arai Y, Kudo K, Hosokawa T, Washio M, Miura H, Hisamichi S. Reliability and validity of the Japanese version of the Zarit Caregiver Burden Interview. Psychiatry Clin Neurosci. 1997;51:281–7.
53. McConaghy R, Caltabiano ML. Caring for a person with dementia: exploring relationships between perceived burden, depression, coping and well-being. Nurs Health Sci. 2005;7:81–91.
54. Washio M, Arai Y, Oura A, et al. Care burden and depression among caregivers of the frail elderly with home-visiting nursing service before and after the introduction of the public long-term care insurance for the elderly: the findings from the studies until the fifth year of the insurance system. Rinsho To Kenkyu. 2005;82:1366–70. (in Japanese)
55. Ogino H, Toyoshima Y, Haruna S, Moriyama H, Matsuda S, Washio M. Factors related to a heavy burden among family caregivers of the frail elderly who use home-visit nursing care services in rural area of the Tokai region. Rinsho To Kenkyu. 2017;94(12):1557–62. (in Japanese)
56. Portal Site of Official Statistics of Japan (e-Stat). Number of clients who use home-visiting nursing care, details of nursing services in September, degree of need of care. In: Ministry of health, labour and welfare. National survey of nursing-care service facilities; 2017. (in Japanese). http://www.estat.go.jp. Accessed 06 Dec 2017.
57. Hashimoto K, Sato K, Uchiumi J, et al. Current home palliative care for terminally ill cancer patients in Japan. Palliat Care Res. 2015;10(1):153–61. (in Japanese)
58. Ishi Y, Miyashita M, Sato K, Ozawa T. Difficulties in caring for terminal cancer patients at home: family caregivers' and homecare providers' perspectives. Nihon Gan Kango Gakkaishi. 2011;25(1):24–36. (in Japanese)
59. Health and Welfare Statistics Association. Trend of national health 2000. Tokyo: Health and Welfare Statistics Association; 2000. (in Japanese)
60. Health and Welfare Statistics Association. Trend of national health 2004. Tokyo: Health and Welfare Statistics Association; 2004. (in Japanese)
61. Health and Welfare Statistics Association. Trend of national health 2010–2011. Tokyo: Health and Welfare Statistics Association; 2010. (in Japanese)

Chapter 3
Health Promotion and Long-Term Care for the Elderly in Rural Areas of Hokkaido, Japan

Mitsuru Mori, Kazutoshi Kitazawa, Satoko Showa, Miki Takeuchi, Toshiaki Seko, and Shunichi Ogawa

Abstract There is a pressing necessity to find an effective means of health promotion, especially, in rural areas of Hokkaido Prefecture, in which local residents themselves can be actively involved. Several epidemiological studies have thus been conducted to grasp a feasible way of promoting health in the area. We found, from the time-series study measured with an accelerometer in Hokkaido, that the average number of step counts, the averages of total energy consumption per day and energy consumption by physical activity per day, and the average duration of moderate and vigorous physical activity were all significantly less in the snowfall season than the non-snowfall season. Therefore, a light-burden and indoor physical exercise program called "Fumanet" exercise, or net-step exercise (NSE), has been developed. From the result of a longitudinal study conducted in Hokkaido, the elderly who participated in NSE classes once a month or more had a significantly lower risk of poor self-rated health 2 years after their participation, compared with nonparticipants. Furthermore, from a result of an 8-week intervention study in Hokkaido, we found that cognitive function assessed by the Touch-M test and gait performance assessed by the Timed Up and Go test were significantly improved by participation in NSE classes among healthy older adults. Our results indicate that NSE offers an option for the older population whose maintenance of cognitive health and gait function require easier methods. In other words, such NSE classes are a feasible method for older people's health promotion in lesser populated municipalities.

Keywords Health promotion · Elderly · Physical activity

M. Mori (✉) · T. Seko · S. Ogawa
Hokkaido Chitose College of Rehabilitation, Chitose, Hokkaido, Japan
e-mail: m-mori@chitose-reha.ac.jp

K. Kitazawa · S. Showa
Non-Profit Organization for Fumanet, Sapporo, Hokkaido, Japan

M. Takeuchi
Can-nus Kushiro, Association of National Volunteer Nurses, Hamanaka-cho, Hokkaido, Japan

3.1   Recommendation of the Net-Step Exercise (NSE) for Health Promotion Among the Elderly in Rural Areas of Hokkaido

There are four seasons in Hokkaido Prefecture, which is located in the northern part of Japan. It snows in winter, and it is thought that as a result of this, physical activity decreases. Consequently, we conducted a time-series study to assess reduction in physical activity in winter (unpublished work), and the results of this study are shown in part in Sect. 3.2.

There are numerous rural areas with low population in Hokkaido. In such areas, health-care services and health science authorities are limited. Accordingly, there is an increased need for an effective means of health promotion in which local residents themselves can be actively involved. Although there is a reasonable number of evidence that higher physical activity promotes individual health, it is necessary to consider forms of physical activity that are easy to perform and less physically burdensome, especially, for the elderly.

Therefore, a light-burden and indoor physical exercise program called "Fumanet" exercise has been developed in Hokkaido [1, 2]. Fumanet is derived from "net" and *fumanai* which in Japanese means to avoid stepping on something. Fumanet is a 4 m × 1.5 m net that is comprised of 50 cm × 50 cm squares arranged in a 3 × 8 grid (Fig. 3.1). One or two persons at a time are required to walk carefully, yet rhythmically, from one end of the Fumanet to the other without stepping on the ropes or being caught in the net. NSE is conducted with groups of approximately ten people each. In this paper, Fumanet exercise is abbreviated to the net-step exercise (NSE). NSE requires the simultaneous use of cognitive function and gait performance.

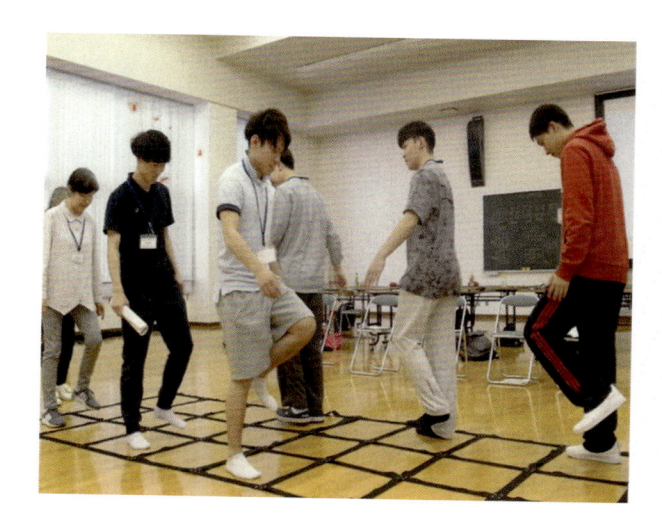

Fig. 3.1 Photograph of Fumanet exercise or the net-step exercise (NSE)

Results of a longitudinal study and an intervention study on effectiveness of NSE are shown in part in Sects. 3.3 and 3.4, respectively [1, 2].

3.2 Time-Series Study on Reduction in Physical Activity in the Snowfall Season Among the Elderly in Chitose, Hokkaido

3.2.1 Introduction

It has been suggested that the climate and other environmental factors may influence physical activity, and there is large diversity in physical activity among different climates [3–7]. However, studies on the differences in physical activity among seasons are few, to our knowledge, even in the snowfall area. Therefore, we examined seasonal differences in physical activity in the daily life of the elderly, comparing physical activity in the snowfall season with that in the non-snowfall season in Chitose, Hokkaido.

3.2.2 Methods

Chitose is located in the central-western part of Hokkaido and had a population of 96,428 in 2015. We recruited study subjects from adults aged 50 years or older who had participated in the health promotion program provided by Chitose office. We excluded persons who had difficulty in understanding the measurement contents, as well as those who had been diagnosed as having a psychiatric disorder, orthopedic disease, stroke, or disorder with severe pain. A total of 35 subjects (12 males, 23 females) participated in this study, after excluding three subjects due to fitting the exclusion criteria. Written informed consent under full explanation about the study was obtained from each study subject.

Their physical activity was measured with an accelerometer, i.e., the Kenz Lifecorder GS (Suzuken Co. Ltd., Nagoya). Items measured with this device were as follows: the number of step counts (STEP) per day, total energy consumption (TEA) per day (kcal), energy consumption by physical activity (ECPA) per day (kcal), and duration (min) of moderate and vigorous physical activity (MVPA). TEA per day is figured out as summation of ECPA per day and energy consumption by basic metabolism per day.

The Kenz Lifecorder GS is utilized via attachment to the waist of a person. It is advised to use from the time getting up to the time going to bed, excluding bathing time, and live as routine a life as possible. We adopted the previously proposed criteria for a sufficiently worn day as wearing it more than or equal to 10 h [8, 9].

Table 3.1 Comparison of background characteristics and physical activity in 35 study subjects and weather conditions of Chitose between the snowfall and the non-snowfall seasons (Ogawa et al. in subm.) (Mean ± standard deviation)

Variable	Snowfall season	Non-snowfall season	Difference in absolute value	P value
STEP	6420 ± 3098	8127 ± 3677	1707 ± 2439	<0.001
TEA (kcal)	1618 ± 148	1682 ± 195	64 ± 112	0.002
ECPA (kcal)	182 ± 82	236 ± 115	47 ± 65	<0.001
MVPA (min)	17 ± 15	22 ± 22	6 ± 11	0.007
Temperature (°C)	−4.1 ± 3.9	17.0 ± 2.4	21.2 ± 0.8	<0.001
Wind velocity (m)	3.6 ± 1.7	3.1 ± 1.0	0.5 ± 0.6	0.117
Precipitation (mm)	– (Not applicable)	6.0 ± 20.0		
Snowfall (cm)	2.6 ± 4.5	– (Not applicable)		

STEP average number of step counts per day, *TEA* average of total energy consumption per day, *ECPA* average of energy consumption by physical activity per day, *MVPA* average duration of moderate and vigorous physical activity per day (min)

The survey was conducted both in September 2015 for the non-snowfall season and in February 2016 for the snowfall season.

3.2.3 Results

The average age (standard deviation, SD) of the 35 study subjects was 69.3 (5.3) years, and means (SDs) of body height, body weight, and body mass index (BMI) were 155.8 (6.5) cm, 56.2 (7.3) kg, and 23.2 (2.7) kg/m², respectively. As shown in Table 3.1, the average number of step counts (STEP) was significantly less in the snowfall season (6420) than in the non-snowfall season (8127), and the difference was 1707 ($p < 0.001$). Similarly, the average of total energy consumption (TEA) per day was significantly less in the snowfall season (1618 kcal) than in the non-snowfall season (1682 kcal), and the difference was 64 kcal ($p = 0.002$). The average of energy consumption by physical activity (ECPA) per day was also significantly less in the snowfall season (182 kcal) than in the non-snowfall season (236 kcal), and the difference was 47 kcal ($p < 0.001$). In addition, the average duration of moderate and vigorous physical activity (MVPA) was significantly shorter in the snowfall season (17 min) than in the non-snowfall season (22 min), and the difference was 6 min ($p = 0.007$). The average temperature (standard deviation) of the snowfall and non-snowfall seasons in Chitose was −4.1 °C (3.9) and 17.0 °C (2.4), respectively ($p < 0.001$). There was no difference in average wind velocity between the snowfall (3.6 m) and the non-snowfall seasons (3.1 m) in Chitose.

3.2.4 Discussion

Physical activities such as STEP, TEA, ECPA, and MVPA measured with an accelerometer were found to be significantly less in the snowfall season than the non-snowfall season. Togo et al. [4] reported that the step count increased with the mean ambient temperature over the range of -2–17 °C but decreased over the range of 17–29 °C. Yasunaga et al. [5] conducted a survey of Japanese elderly aged 65–83 years, using an accelerometer, and, similar to our study, they showed that step counts and amounts of physical activity were low in the winter, peaking in spring and autumn. Wagner et al. [7] examined the association between weather conditions and outdoor exercise with a survey using a structured questionnaire and found that the study subjects delayed outdoor exercise in winter, compared with other seasons.

The daily step counts are recommended to be more than 8000, and the daily duration of MVPA is recommended to be more than 20 min (150 min per week) by Aoyagi and Shephard [10]. Average physical activities of our study subjects were observed to be above the recommended levels in the non-snowfall season; however, they were below the recommended levels in the snowfall season.

There are several limitations in our study. Firstly, because of the small sample size in our study, examining a larger number of study subjects would be required in future studies. Secondly, because the study subjects may be relatively healthier, it is not possible to generalize our results to all adults living in the snowfall area. Thirdly, since we did not include a sufficient number of lifestyle or psychological factors in our study, it is necessary to consider those factors in the future study. Fourthly, although physical activity was measured with one axial accelerometer in our study, the devise mentions that the measurement accuracy is low when conducting less-intensive activity such as housework. A three-axial accelerometer would be recommended for future studies because of the higher accuracy in the less-intensive activity [11].

3.2.5 Conclusion

Through the time-series study measured with an accelerometer, it was discovered that the average number of step counts (STEP), the average of total energy consumption (TEA) per day, the average of energy consumption by physical activity (ECPA), and duration of moderate and vigorous physical activity (MVPA) were all significantly less in the snowfall season than the non-snowfall season.

3.3 Longitudinal Study on the Influence of Participation in Net-Step Exercise (NSE) Class for Elderly in Ikeda, Hokkaido

3.3.1 Introduction

We conducted a longitudinal study to assess the influence of participation in classes of Fumanet exercise or NSE among older residents in Ikeda, Hokkaido [2]. Ikeda is located in the central-eastern part of Hokkaido and is recognized as one of the lesser populated areas. The population of Ikeda was 7572 in 2012, and the proportion of the elderly aged 65 years or over was 35.4%. Residents have relatively frequently held NSE classes in Ikeda, and a proportion of participants in NSE have been among the highest in Hokkaido. Self-rated health (SHR) was used for the outcome variable because SHR has been shown to be significantly predicting for all-cause mortality [12, 13].

3.3.2 Methods

For a cohort consisting of 666 participants developed in 2012 in Ikeda, a follow-up survey was conducted in 2014. Written informed consent was obtained from each subject. In surveys regarding NSE participation at the time of baseline, the following question was posed to the participants: "In the last year, how many times did you participate in NSE per month on average?" The participants chose their response from four options (never; 1–2 times monthly; 3–4 times monthly; or at least 5 times monthly), and their answer was 75.5%, 14.5%, 3.8%, and 6.2%, respectively. A comparison was made between those who answered never (500 subjects) and those who answered more than or equal to once a month (166 subjects).

Self-rated health (SRH) was surveyed at the time of follow-up using the following question: "Overall, how was your health condition in the past month on average?" The participants chose their response from the following six options: extremely good, very good, good, not very good, not good, and not good at all. A comparison was made between good SRH (answered as extremely good, very good, or good) and poor SHR (answered as not very good, not good, or not good at all). Analysis with the multivariable logistic regression model was applied to calculate an odds ratio (OR) with 95% confidence interval (CI) for the association between participation in the NSE class and poor SRH.

3.3.3 Results

As shown in Table 3.2, the age- and sex-adjusted OR of participation in NSE classes more than or equal to once a month at baseline against poor SRH 2 years later at the follow-up was 0.53 (95% CI 0.34–0.78). After adjusting for age, sex, and other

Table 3.2 Odds ratio (OR) with 95% confidence interval (CI) of poor self-rated health in follow-up related to net-step exercise (NSE) participation in baseline (Showa et al. 2016)

Variable	Content	Number of subjects	Age- and sex-adjusted OR (95% CI)	Multivariable- adjusted OR (95% CI)#
NSE participation	None	500	1.00	1.00
	≥once per month	166	0.49 (0.30–0.78)	0.50 (0.29–0.85)

#Age, sex, education level, living arrangement, and regular exercise were adjusted

potential confounding variables, such as education level, living arrangement, and regular exercise, the adjusted OR was 0.50 (95% CI 0.29–0.85), which was significant as well.

3.3.4 Discussion

This study revealed that NSE class participation provided by the residents was inversely associated with poor SRH in older people 2 years after participation. This result is consistent with previous studies, which showed association of physical activity with decreased risk of poor SRH [14–17]. From the result of the follow-up study, Malmberg et al. [14] reported that no weekly vigorous global leisure time activity was associated with an increased risk of decline in SRH in men. From the result of the cross-sectional study, Han et al. [15] discerned that the prevalence of poor SRH was significantly lower as the level of physical activity increased. Wang et al. [16] found from a result of the cross-sectional study that a lack in physical activity had a strong positive association with poor SRH both in men and women.

In addition, our study might support previous studies of significant association between more social participation and better SRH [18–20]. Fujiwara et al. [18] reported that elderly volunteers who read books for children during the 18 months significantly improved their SRH compared with the control group. Nieminen et al. [20] showed from a result of the cross-sectional study that good SRH was associated with a high level of social participation.

There are several limitations in this study. Firstly, the cohort was limited to 56% of the population. Secondly, the one-time assessment of NSE class participation excluded the opportunity to account for the later changes in NSE class participation. Thirdly, data on some potential confounding factors, such as socioeconomic status and mental health, were unavailable in this study.

3.3.5 Conclusion

From the result of a longitudinal study, the older individuals who participated in NSE classes once a month or more had a significantly lower risk of poor SRH 2 years after their participation compared with class nonparticipants. Such NSE classes are a feasible method for older people's health promotion in municipalities with a lower population.

3.4 Intervention Study on Effects of the Net-Step Exercise (NSE) for Elderly in Kushiro, Hokkaido

3.4.1 Introduction

Physical activity has been shown to have a beneficial effect on cognitive function and reduce the risks of dementia [21–24]. In addition, physical activity has a beneficial effect on gait performance and reduces the risk of falls [24]. There is an increased need to identify types and levels of physical activity that are suitable for the majority of older people to improve their cognitive function and gait performance [25]. Our study aimed to assess the effect of a light-burden NSE performed once a week for eight consecutive weeks on improvement in cognitive function and gait performance [1].

3.4.2 Methods

A randomized single-blind controlled trial was used to evaluate the effect of the NSE on cognitive and gait function in older adults in 2014. Participants included volunteers from the federation of senior citizen's club in Kushiro, located in the eastern area of Hokkaido. The participants had to possess a driver's license and drive more than once a week, in order to exclude individuals with dementia or other cognitive and physical impairments. In Japan, driver's license holders whom are older than 70 years must pass an official government screening test for dementia, eyesight, and motor skills every 3 years.

Thus, 60 participants between the ages of 71 and 89 years were enrolled in the study. Written informed consent was obtained from each subject. Participants were randomly assigned into the NSE group (30 persons) and the control group (30 persons) using a lottery. The 8-week NSE program was conducted at the same time and day of the week and in the same room at Hokkaido University of Education, Kushiro Campus, for all members of the intervention group. Throughout the 8-week NSE program, the difficulty of the step designs and the number of steps required in each session were gradually increased. Participants walked 216 steps per session during the first 4 weeks of the program and 240 steps per session for the fifth and eighth.

Cognitive assessment was conducted using a device with a touch-panel computer screen called the Touch-M system [26]. The Touch-M system evaluates visuospatial function in the lateral prefrontal area to assess cognitive function and diagnose early stages of Alzheimer disease. The Touch-M system runs on the Microsoft Windows operating system and a touch-panel-type desktop PC.

The Timed Up and Go (TUG) test was used to measure gait performance. The TUG test requires the subject to stand up, walk 3 m, turn, walk back, and sit down, and the time (min) taken to complete the TUG is measured [27]. The repeated measures procedure was used in an analysis of covariance (ANCOVA). The two time points (baseline and 8 weeks) were treated as a within-participant factor. The difference between the NSE and control groups was treated as a between-participant factor. Covariates, such as age and sex, were included in the multivariate model.

3.4.3   Results

As shown in Table 3.3, the total score of the Touch-M test significantly improved by 5.4 points from the baseline in the NSE group ($p = 0.04$), and the mean difference from the baseline in the Touch-M test score was 4.9 times higher in the NSE group compared with the control group ($p = 0.04$). The time in the TUG test significantly improved by 0.98 s in the NSE group relative to the baseline assessment, and the results from the repeated measures ANCOVA showed a significant effect for the within-participant interaction in the TUG test ($p < 0.001$).

3.4.4   Discussion

Our study demonstrated that the NSE group had significant improvement of cognitive function after 8 weeks of NSE. This finding is consistent with previous research. Larson et al. [21] found from a result of the cohort study that persons who exercised three times or more per week had a reduced hazard ratio for developing dementia compared with those who exercised fewer than three times per week. Lautenschlarger et al. [22] reported from the result of a randomized controlled trial that participants in the physical activity group had better scores of cognitive function than those in the control group.

Table 3.3 Effect of the net-step exercise on gait and cognitive function in participants at the end of 8 weeks (Kitazawa et al. 2015)

Test	Mean difference from baseline with 95% confidence interval		P value for repeated measures ANCOVA	
	NSE group ($n = 30$)	Control group ($n = 30$)	Between participants	Within participants
Touch-M score in total	5.40 (2.29 to 8.51)	1.10 (−1.43 to 3.63)	0.04	0.04
Timed Up and Go test	−0.98 (−1.34 to −0.61)	0.40 (−0.01 to 0.81)	0.33	<0.001

ANCOVA, analysis of covariance

Our study also showed that gait performance was significantly improved in the NSE group compared with the control group. Similar to our result, Shubert et al. [24] reported from an intervention study that participants in exercise-based balance improvement program showed a significant improvement in gait performance. Moreover, cognitive function has been shown to be an indicator of gait and balance performance [28–30]. From this point of view, it is also assumed that NSE simultaneously improves cognitive function and gait performance.

This study has some limitations. Firstly, because a double-blinded study design was not possible, it was inevitable that participants discovered whether they belonged to the intervention or control groups. Secondly, the physical activity and social activity of the participants other than NSE were not controlled or monitored. Thirdly, potential confounding factors, such as socioeconomic status and lifestyle, were not included in this study.

3.4.5   Conclusion

From the result of the 8-week intervention study, we found that cognitive function, assessed by the Touch-M test, and gait performance, assessed by the Timed Up and Go (TUG) test, were significantly improved by participation in NSE classes among healthy older adults. Our results indicate that NSE offers an option for a large segment of the older population who require an easier way to maintain their cognitive health and gait function.

3.5   Future Study Planning

More than 6000 elderly individuals have been registered as NSE supporters by obtaining the qualified training of FSE in Hokkaido. There are some rural areas which are abundant in the NSE supporters, as well as in NSE participants. Accordingly, a longitudinal study of NSE supporters and NSE participants, as well as nonparticipants, is now undergoing planning to examine the effectiveness of NSE with a lager sample size in such areas.

References

1. Kitazawa K, Showa S, Hiraoka A, et al. Effect of a dual-task net-step exercise on cognitive and gait function in older adults. J Geriatr Phys Ther. 2015;38:133–40.
2. Showa S, Kitazawa K, Takeuchi M, et al. Influence of volunteer-led net step exercise class on older people's self-rated health in a depopulated town: a longitudinal study. SSM Popul Health. 2016;2:130–40.

3. Merrill RM, Shields EC, White GL Jr, et al. Climate conditions and physical activity in the United States. Am J Health Behav. 2005;29:371–81.
4. Togo F, Watanabe E, Park H, et al. Meteorology and the physical activity of the elderly: the Nakanojo study. Int J Biometeorol. 2005;50:83–9.
5. Yasunaga A, Togo F, Watanabe E, et al. Sex, age, season, and habitual physical activity of older Japanese: the Nakanojo study. J Aging Phys Act. 2008;16:3–13.
6. Mizumoto A, Ihira H, Makino K, et al. Physical activity changes in the winter in older persons living in northern Japan: a prospective study. BMC Geriatr. 2015;15:43.
7. Wagner AL, Keusch F, Yan T, et al. The impact of weather on summer and winter exercise behaviors. J Sport Health Sci. 2016; https://doi.org/10.1016/j.jshs.2016.07.0077.
8. Mâsse LC, Fuemmeler BF, Anderson CB, et al. Accelerometer data reduction: a comparison of four reduction algorithms on select outcome variables. Med Sci Sports Exerc. 2005;37:S544–54.
9. Edwardson CL, Gorely T. Epoch length and its effect on physical activity intensity. Med Sci Sports Exerc. 2010;42:928–34.
10. Aoyagi Y, Shephard RJ. Habitual physical activity and health in the elderly: the Nakanojo study. Geriatr Gerontol Int. 2010;10(Suppl 1):S236–43.
11. Ohkawara K, Oshima Y, Hikihara Y, et al. Real-time estimation of daily physical activity intensity by a triaxial accelerometer and a gravity-removal classification algorithm. Br J Nutr. 2011;105:1681–91.
12. Tsuji I, Minami Y, Keyl PM, et al. The predictive power of self-rated health, activities of daily living, and ambulatory activity for cause-specific mortality among the elderly: a three-year follow-up in urban Japan. J Am Geriatr Soc. 2004;42:153–6.
13. Ishizaki T, Kai I, Imanaka Y. Self-rated health and social role as predictors for 6-year total mortality among a non-disabled older Japanese population. Arch Gerontol Geriatr. 2006;42:91–9.
14. Malmberg J, Miilunpalo S, Pasanen M, et al. Characteristics of leisure time physical activity associated with risk of decline in perceived health - a 10-year follow-up of middle aged and elderly men and women. Prev Med. 2005;41:141–50.
15. Han MA, Kim KS, Park J, et al. Association between levels of physical activity and poor self-rated health in Korean adults: the third Korea National Health and nutrition examination survey (KNHANES), 2005. Public Health. 2009;123:665–9.
16. Wang N, Iwasaki M, Otani T, et al. Perceived health as related to income, socio-economic status, lifestyle, and social support factors in a middle-aged Japanese. J Epidemiol. 2005;15:155–62.
17. Cimarras-Otal C, Calderòn-Larrañaga A, Poblador-Plou B, et al. Association between physical activity, multimorbidity, self-rated health and functional limitation in the Spanish population. BMC Public Health. 2014;14:1170.
18. Fujiwara Y, Sakuma N, Ohba H, et al. REPRINTS: effects of an intergenerational health promotion program for older adults in Japan. J Intergender Relatsh. 2009;7:17–39.
19. Hong SI, Morrow-Howell N. Health outcomes of experience corps: a high-commitment volunteer program. Soc Sci Med. 2010;71:414–20.
20. Nieminen T, Martelin T, Koskinen S, et al. Social capital as a determinant of self-rated health and psychological well-being. Int J Public Health. 2010;55:531–42.
21. Larson EB, Wang L, Bowen JD, et al. Exercise is associated with reduced risk for incident dementia among persons 65 years of age and older. Ann Intern Med. 2006;144:73–81.
22. Lautenschlarger NT, Cox KL, Flicker L, et al. Effect of physical activity on cognitive function in older adults at risk for Alzheimer disease: a randomized trial. JAMA. 2008;300:1027–37.
23. Williamson JD, Espeland M, Kritchevsky SB, et al. Change in cognitive function in a randomized trial of physical activity: results of the lifestyle interventions and independence for elders pilot study. J Gerontol A Biol Sci Med Sci. 2009;64:688–94.
24. Shubert TE, McCulloch K, Hartman M, et al. The effect of cognitive an exercise-based balance intervention on physical and cognitive performance for older adults: a pilot study. J Geriatr Phys Ther. 2010;33:157–64.

25. Logsdon RG, McCurry SM, Pike KC, et al. Making physical activity accessible to older adults with memory loss: a feasibility study. Gerontologist. 2009;49:S94–9.
26. Hatakeyama Y, Sasaki R, Ikeda N, et al. Newly developed task using touch screen device to estimate cognitive function especially visuospatial memory, executive function and processing speed. Psychogeriatrics. 2006;17:655–64.
27. Shumway-Cook A, Brauer S, Woollacott M. Predicting the probability for falls in community-dwelling older adults using the timed up & go test. Phys Ther. 2000;80:896–903.
28. van Iersel MB, Kessels RP, Bloem BR, et al. Executive functions are associated with gait and balance in community-living elderly people. J Gerontol A Biol Sci Med Sci. 2008;63:1344–9.
29. Li KZ, Roudaia E, Lussier M, et al. Benefits of cognitive dual-task training on balance performance in healthy older adults. J Gerontol A Biol Sci Med Sci. 2010;65:1344–52.
30. Verghese J, Mahoney J, Ambrose AF, et al. Effect of cognitive remediation on gait in sedentary seniors. J Gerontol A Biol Sci Med Sci. 2010;65:1338–43.

Chapter 4
Prevention Strategy for Frailty

Hunkyung Kim and Tatsuro Ishizaki

Abstract Frailty is one of the most important concerns regarding our aging population. Frailty includes physical, social, oral, psychological, and cognitive aspects due to multisystem declines in physiologic reserve, rendering older adults vulnerable to increased risk of functional disability, falls, hospitalization, long-term care, morbidity, and mortality. Therefore, prevention and treatment of frailty is very important to prolong independence in elderly people. There are numerous factors that contribute to muscle weakness, slow walking speed, and loss of muscle mass in aging adults such as chronic disease, a sedentary lifestyle, and undernutrition, where some factors can be reversed with lifestyle changes and others need specific medications and cannot be reversed. Exercise and nutritional supplementation are among the beneficial treatments promoting healthy and independent lifestyles in the elderly. Evidence reveals that exercise targeted at reducing risk factors is an effective strategy for preventing and/or treating frailty in elderly people. Progressive and moderate-intensity exercise alone or combined with nutritional and hormone supplementation should be encouraged among elderly people to minimize the degenerative physical, psychological, social, and cognitive function that occurs with aging.

Keywords Frailty · Prevention · Treatment · Exercise · Nutrition

4.1 Introduction

Physical, psychological, cognitive, and social function changes occur with aging, and frailty is one of the most important concerns regarding our aging population.

Physical frailty due to multisystem declines in physiologic reserve is common among older adults, rendering them vulnerable to increased risk of functional disability, falls, hospitalization, long-term care, morbidity, and mortality [1–3].

Even though several operational definitions of frailty were proposed to help develop screening criteria, there is not yet a standardized and valid method of clini-

H. Kim (✉) · T. Ishizaki
Tokyo Metropolitan Institute of Gerontology, Tokyo, Japan
e-mail: kimhk@tmig.or.jp

© Springer Nature Singapore Pte Ltd. 2019
M. Washio, C. Kiyohara (eds.), *Health Issues and Care System for the Elderly*,
Current Topics in Environmental Health and Preventive Medicine,
https://doi.org/10.1007/978-981-13-1762-0_4

cal screening for frailty. Despite a lack of international consensus on the definition of frailty, the most commonly used definitions of frailty are the frailty phenotype [3], the frailty index [4], the classification of frailty and vigorousness [5], and the Edmonton frail scale [6]. Among them, Fried's cardiovascular health study (CHS) criteria are the most widely used. Fried et al. proposed the frailty phenotype and described it based on five indicators of physical components: unintentional weight loss, muscle weakness, exhaustion, slow gait speed, and low physical activity. Subjects are considered robust (no criteria present), prefrail (one or two criteria present), or frail (three to five criteria present) [3]. Several other commonly used criteria have modified Fried's frailty phenotype including the Women's Health and Aging Studies (WHAS) [7] and the Japanese version of the CHS [8] (Table 4.1).

Table 4.1 Frailty-defining criteria: Women's Health and Aging Studies (WHAS), Cardiovascular Health Study (CHS), and Japanese version of CHS

Characteristics	CHS	WHAS	Japanese version of CHS
Weight loss	*Baseline:* Lost >10 pounds unintentionally in last year *Follow-up:* (weight in previous year-current weight)/(weight in previous year) ≥0.05 and the loss was unintentional	*Baseline: Either of:* (1) (weight at age 60 – weight at exam)/(weight at age 60) ≥0.1 (2) BMI at exam <18.5 *Follow-up: Either of:* (1) BMI at exam <18.5 (2) (weight in previous year-current weight)/(weight in previous year) ≥0.05 and the loss was unintentional	Have you lost 2 kg or more in the past 6 months? Yes = 1, No = 0
Exhaustion	*Self-report of either of:* (1) Felt that everything I did was an effort in the last week (2) Could not get going in the last week	*Self-report of any of:* (1) Low usual energy level 1 (≤3, range 0–10) (2) Felt unusually tired in the last 2 months (3) Felt unusually weak in the past 2 months	In the past 2 weeks, have you felt tired without a reason? Yes = 1, No = 0
Low physical activity	Based on the short version of Minnesota Leisure Time Activity questionnaire: *Women:* Those with Kcals per week < 270 are frail *Men:* Those with Kcals of physical activity per week < 383 are frail	Women: Kcal <90 on activity scale (6 items) Men: Kcal <128 on activity scale (6 items)	(1) Do you engage in moderate levels of physical exercise or sports aimed at health? (2) Do you engage in low levels of physical exercise aimed at health? "No" to both questions = 1, others = 0

Table 4.1 (continued)

Characteristics	CHS	WHAS	Japanese version of CHS

Slowness	Walk time, stratified by gender and height. Cutoff for Time to Walk 15 feet (4.57m) criteria for frailty
	Women:
	  time >= 7 seconds for height <= 159 cm
	  time >= 6 seconds for height > 159 cm
	Men:
	  time >= 7 seconds for height <= 173 cm
	  time >= 6 seconds for height > 173 cm
		Walking 4 at usual pace
		Women:
		  speed ≤4.57/7 meter/ seconds for height ≤159 cm
		  speed ≤4.57/6 meter/ seconds for height >159 cm
		Men:
		  speed ≤4.57/7 meter/ seconds for height ≤173 cm
		  speed ≤4.57/6 meter/ seconds for height >173 cm
			Gait speed <1.0 meter/ seconds

Weakness	Grip strength, stratified by gender and BMI quartiles. Cutoff for grip strength criteria for frailty
	Women:
	  <= 17 kg for BMI <= 23
	  <=17.3 kg for BMI 23.1–26
	  <= 18 kg for BMI 26.1–29
	  <= 21 kg for BMI > 29
	Men:
	  <= 29 kg for BMI <= 24
	  <= 30 kg for BMI 24.1–26
	  <= 30 kg for BMI 26.1–28
	  <= 32 kg for BMI > 28
		Grip strength: Same as in CHS	Grip strength
			  Men: <26 kg
			  Women: <18 kg

Notes: *BMI* body mass index (kg/m²)

Recently, there have been trends toward classifying frailty into physical, psychological, cognitive, and social aspects; however, a standardized definition has not been established (Fig. 4.1) [9]. The CHS criteria are technically used for physical frailty. In this chapter, the focus will be placed on definitions within the more established physical frailty.

Depending on the frailty definition and evaluation tool, frailty prevalence ranges between 4.0% and 59.1% in community-dwelling people aged 65 years [10]. As the population ages, frailty represents increasingly important public health concerns and has an incremental effect on health expenditures [11]. Because of the major clinical, long-term care and economic burden, it is critical to find efficient, feasible, and cost-effective interventions to prevent or slow down frailty in order to avoid or diminish the adverse health outcomes, maintain or improve quality of life, and reduce disability and extended healthy life expectancy [12].

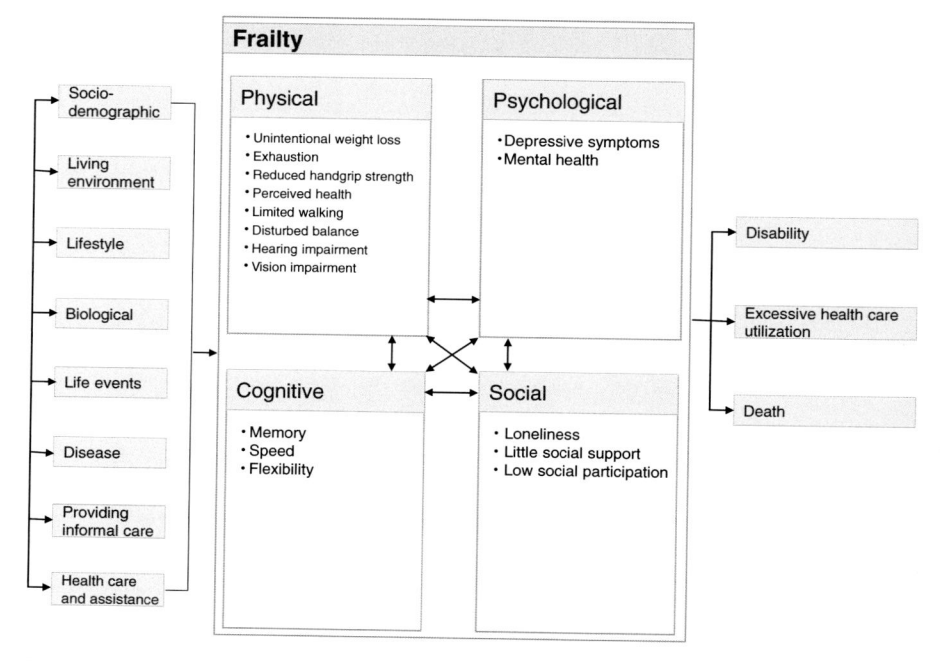

Fig. 4.1 Adapted version of integral conceptual model of frailty (cited from reference 9 published by BioMed Central)

4.2 Risk Factors

There are numerous factors that contribute to muscle weakness and loss of muscle mass in aging adults such as chronic disease, a sedentary lifestyle, and undernutrition, where some factors can be reversed with lifestyle changes and others need specific medications and cannot be reversed. Xue et al. hypothesized the cycle of frailty, as many of these factors can theoretically be unified into a cycle associated with decreasing energetics and functional reserve (Fig. 4.2). The core elements of this cycle, including weight loss, sarcopenia, decrease in strength and walking speed, as well as low activity, are commonly identified as clinical signs and symptoms of frailty [13].

4.3 Prevention Strategy

Declines in functional fitness such as walking speed and muscle strength and low physical activity in the elderly are strongly associated with the development of frailty. Hence, exercise and nutritional supplementation focusing on strength and mobility improvement, and physical activity increment even into advanced age, is usually offered as a strategy for the prevention and/or reduction of frailty in the elderly. Further, investigation into disability risk with each frailty criterion showed

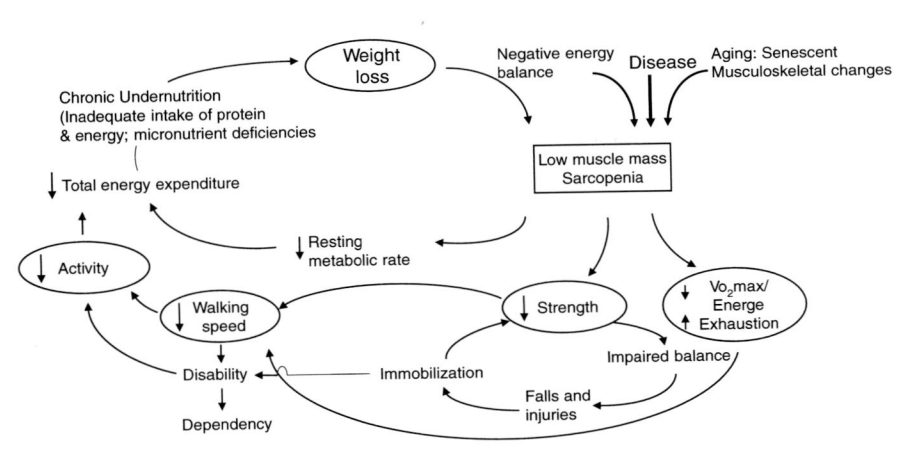

Fig. 4.2 Cycle of frailty [13] (Xue QL, Bandeen-Roche K, Varadhan R, Zhou J, & Fried LP (2008). Initial manifestations of frailty criteria and the development of frailty phenotype in the Women's Health and Aging Study II. The Journals of Gerontology. Series A, Biological Sciences and Medical Sciences, Vol 63A, No9, pp 984–990, by permission of Oxford University Press)

that declines in walking speed (HR = 2.32, 95% CI = 1.62–3.33), muscle strength decline (HR = 1.90, 95% CI = 1.35–2.68), and weight loss (HR = 1.61, 95% CI = 1.13–2.31) were most strongly associated with disability [14]. These findings show that frailty prevention should focus not only on walking ability and muscle strength but preventing unintentional weight loss as well. Out of many factors related with frailty, muscle disuse and nutritional deficiencies are potentially reversible or preventable through interventions and changes in lifestyle.

4.3.1 Nutritional Supplementation

Declines in muscle mass are related to declines in muscle protein synthesis rates in older adults. In order to resist and reverse the effects of muscle protein synthesis declines, protein or, more specifically, amino acids have been the focus of research. Investigators have found that leucine-enriched essential amino acid mixtures are primarily responsible for amino acid-induced muscle protein anabolism in the elderly. Amino acid supplementation can increase muscle mass in this population; however, an increase in muscle mass is not always accompanied by an increase in muscle strength [15]. Essential amino acid supplementation alone is probably insufficient in increasing muscle strength. Carbohydrate-rich supplements have also been examined for any effects on muscle strength and muscle mass. However, supplements rich in carbohydrates are inadequate for increasing muscle mass and strength [16]. There has been a peaked interest in other nutritional supplementations including protein, tea catechins, vitamin D, omega-3 fatty acids, and MFGM (milk fat globule membrane), as their efficacy in improving muscle mass and strength have been reported.

4.3.2 Exercise

There are several systematic reviews published on the benefits of exercise in frail elderly adults. Exercise in these individuals may potentially modify risk factors for age-associated reductions in muscle mass [17]. Research has shown that high-intensity resistance training is effective in counteracting muscle weakness and physical frailty in elderly people. Exercise interventions focusing on the major muscle groups that are crucial for performing functional activities are especially important for the reversal of muscle weakness.

Extensive research has confirmed that doing resistance training two to three times a week can improve physical function and functional limitations and also reduce disability and muscle weakness in older people. Resistance training in elderly people produces increases in strength from 9% to 15% [18] and about 1.1 kg in lean body mass [19]. More improvements are seen with high-intensity and high-volume resistance training. However, moderate-intensity exercises are also beneficial and are much safer for aging adults. Exercise prescriptions must be of a safe intensity, duration, and frequency to avoid further injury and complications [20].

4.3.3 Combination

Combinations of both exercise and nutritional supplementation have also been studied by researchers. Amino acid supplementations alone have beneficial effects such as increasing walking speed, and exercise, as we have previously seen, has beneficial effects of improving physical function as well. Exercise and amino acid supplementation together have significant effects in enhancing muscle mass, strength, and functional fitness [21]. The combination of high-resistance exercise and a high-carbohydrate mixture containing small amounts of soy protein is effective in the enhancement of muscle strength. High-resistance exercise alone increases both muscle mass and strength, while the carbohydrate supplementation alone does not [16]. In order to efficiently prevent frailty, more focus should be placed on eliminating variable factors within risk factors. Recent studies have shown that the combination of exercise and nutritional supplementation is more effective than exercise or nutrition alone.

4.4 Treatment Strategy

Exercise programs designed for frailty prevention and/or treatment in elderly people should address three major components – strength, gait, and muscle mass. People at high risk of frailty due to muscle weakness, gait deficit, and skeletal muscle mass decline should be instructed to perform low- or moderate-intensity exercise containing safe and simple movements at entry level.

In 2017, Dedyne et al. performed a systematic review to determine the effects of comprehensive intervention programs on the treatment of prefrailty and frailty [22]. A multi-domain intervention was defined as one that intervenes in at least two different domains, including exercise therapy, nutritional intervention (supplementation of proteins, vitamins, minerals, milk fat globule membrane, or nutritional advice), hormone supplementation, cognitive training, or psychosocial interventions. The review included 5500 studies published by September 14, 2016, with inclusion criteria as follows: (1) randomized controlled trials, quasi-experimental studies, or prospective or retrospective cohort studies with control groups, (2) testing of a multi-domain intervention to prevent or treat frailty in people aged, $\geq$65 years, (3) classification in terms of (pre)frailty status according to an operationalized definition, and (4) primary outcomes including one or more of the following – frailty status or score, muscle mass, strength or power, physical functioning, and cognitive or social outcomes. A total of 12 studies matched the criteria. On the other hand, Puts et al. discussed 14 studies found among 14,564 published between January 2000 and February 2016, in a coping review of frailty-related literature [23].

This chapter will provide an overview of some of the main studies within the 26 presented in the two aforementioned reviews (Table 4.2). However, because frailty criteria and main outcome variables differ depending on the publication, providing a comprehensive overview is difficult.

4.4.1 Intervention Characteristics

Although all studies labeled their participants as frail, there were subcategorizations including moderately frail, mild to moderate physical frail, risk of becoming frail, and prefrail. Furthermore, many studies utilized one of the validated operational definitions of frailty: Fried's frailty phenotype [3], Speechley and Tinetti's classification of frailty and vigorousness [5], and Winograd's frailty scale [4]. In other studies, non-validated definitions of frailty were used. There are no standardized universal selection criteria used. These factors should be considered in the following summary of the interventions.

1. Frequency: The greater part of the exercise interventions was performed either twice or three times per week. Several studies increased the exercise frequency to five times or decrease to one time per week.
2. Intensity: In a few studies, the exercise intensity was evaluated using a perceived exertion scale. Most of the interventions that utilized a resistance training program reported intensity as three sets of eight repetitions at approximately 80% of the individual's one repetition maximum (1RM). Several resistance training programs compared low-intensity (20 and 40% 1RM) to high-intensity (80% 1RM) training and found that the changes in muscle strength and endurance were greater in the high-intensity group compared with low-intensity.

Table 4.2 Summary of study characteristics

Study	Country	Study participants	Intervention	Duration	Follow-up	Frequency	N	Frailty diagnostic tool
Chin A Paw et al. [32]	Netherlands	Frail, men and women, aged 78.7 (±5.6 yr)	Exercise: skill training Nutritional: fruit and daily products enriched with vitamin and minerals	17 weeks		2/week 45 min	157	Modified Chin A Paw frailty definition
Hennessey et al. [35]	USA	Moderately frail, men and women, aged 71.3 (±4.5) yr	Exercise: resistance training Growth hormone administration: 0.0025–0.0037 mg/kg/day	6 months		3/week 60 min	31	Physical performance test (PPT): score (12–28)/36
Rydwik et al. [27]	Sweden	Frail, men and women, aged 75+ (yr)	Exercise: aerobic, muscle strength, and balance training Nutritional: individual dietary counseling	12 weeks	6 months	2/week 60 min	96	Modified Chin A Paw frailty definition
Kenny et al. [25]	USA	(Pre) Frail, women, aged 76.6 (±6.0 yr)	Exercise: yoga or chair aerobics Nutritional: calcium and cholecalciferol Hormone: 50 mg/day DHEA	6 months		2/week 90 min	99	At least 1 of 5 Fried frailty criteria: population is at least prefrail
Tieland et al. [24]	Netherlands	(Pre)frail, men and women, aged 78 (±1.0 yr)	Exercise: resistance training Nutritional: 250 mL protein supplemented beverage with 15 g protein	24 weeks		2/week	62	1–2 (prefrail) or at least 3 (frail) of the Fried frailty phenotype criteria
Chan et al. [28]	Taiwan	(Pre)frail, men and women, aged 71.4 (±3.7 yr)	Exercise: resistance, postal control and balance training Nutritional: consultation	3 months	3, 9 months	3/week 60 min	117	3–6 on the Chinese-Canadian Study of Health and Aging Clinical Frailty Scale Telephone version and ≥1 of modified Fried frailty phenotype criteria
Cameron et al. [36]	Australia	Frail, men and women, aged 70+ (yr)	Exercise: home-based balance and mobility improvement training Nutritional: high-energy and high-protein supplements Encourage greater social engagement	3 months	9 months	3–5/week	241	The CHS criteria

Kim et al. [29]	Japan	Frail, women, aged 75+ (yr)	Exercise: comprehensive training Nutritional: milk fat globule membrane (1 g/day)	3 months	4 months	2/week 60 min	131	At least 3 of the modified Fried frailty phenotype criteria
Kwon et al. [33]	Japan	Prefrail, women, aged 70+ (yr)	Exercise: strength training Nutritional: education and cooking classes	3 months	6 months	1/week 60 min	89	Modified Fried frailty phenotype criteria
Ng et al. [34]	Singapore	(Pre)frail, men and women, aged 65+ (yr)	Exercise: home-based strength and balance training Nutritional: iron, folate, vitamin, and calcium supplement Cognitive: cognitive-enhancing activities	6 months	6 months	2/week 90 min	246	Fried frailty phenotype criteria
Luger et al. [38]	Austria	(Pre)frail, men and women, aged 65+ (yr)	Exercise: strength training Nutritional: dietary discussions, fluid intake, animal and plant protein intake, and energy intake	12 weeks		2/week 60 min	80	Prefrail or frail according to Frailty Instrument for Primary Care of the Survey of Health, Ageing, and Retirement in Europe
Tarazona-Santabalbina et al. [30]	Spain	Frail, men and women, aged 70+ (yr)	Exercise: multicomponent exercise (endurance, strength, coordination, balance and flexibility) Nutritional: nutritional information	24 weeks		2/week 60 min	100	Fried frailty phenotype criteria
Ikeda et al. [31]	Japan	(Pre)frail, men and women, aged 78.4 ± 7.8 yr and 80.4 ± 8.9 yr	Exercise: muscle strength and aerobic exercise Nutritional: 6-g amino acid	3 months		2/week	52	Fried frailty phenotype criteria

Notes: *yr* year, *PPT* physical performance test, *CHS* cardiovascular health study

However, improvements for functional ability were only marginally different between the two groups.

3. Duration: The duration of the interventions ranged from 3 to 12 months, and the most common duration was 3 months. The time per session ranged from 45 to 90 min, and the majority of the studies included interventions that lasted 60 min per session.

4. Type: Many of previous studies included multicomponent exercise intervention (usually focusing on resistance, balance, aerobic, and flexibility training), a few resistance training, and some other types of exercise interventions (walking exercise program, balance training, water exercise, tai chi, whole-body vibration exercise, and exercise using a horse-riding simulator).

4.4.2 Changes in the Components of the Frailty Phenotype

Fried et al. [3] described frailty in the Cardiovascular Health Study (CHS). More specifically, the Phenotypic Classification of Frailty (CHS-PCF) [3] includes five components: unintentional weight loss, muscle weakness, exhaustion, slow gait speed, and low physical activity. In the following sections, effects of exercise or nutrition supplementation trials in frail elderly on these components are described with detail.

4.4.2.1 Change in Muscle Mass (Unintentional Weight Loss)

Several studies examined muscle mass after an intervention (Table 4.3). Three studies observed treatment×time interactions. Tieland et al. [24] found that adding a protein and mineral supplementation to resistance exercise at increasing intensity significantly improved appendicular (exercise + protein, 20.1–21.0 kg; exercise + placebo, 19.3–19.1 kg, $P < 0.001$) and lean mass (exercise + protein, 47.2–48.5 kg; exercise + placebo, 45.7–45.4 kg, $P = 0.006$) post-intervention. Kenny et al. [25] found that adding a hormonal dehydroepiandrosterone intervention to an exercise and vitamin and mineral supplementation increased total lean mass post-intervention (exercise + DHEA, 39.6 ± 6.1 kg; exercise + placebo, 38.1 ± 5.2 kg, $P = 0.048$). However, there was no significant change in appendicular muscle mass. de Jong et al. [26] did not find significant changes in the comparison between all four groups, but a factorial analysis of the exercise group ($n = 75$; exercise alone and exercise + nutrition groups) and non-exercise group ($n = 68$; nutrition and control groups) showed significantly improved lean body mass in an exercise intervention combined with a protein, vitamin, and mineral supplementation intervention ($+0.5$ kg, $P = 0.02$) compared to no exercise or protein, vitamin, and mineral supplementation (-0.1 kg, $P = 0.60$). Several other studies also found significant improvements in within-group comparisons although significant interactions were not observed. Rydwik et al. [27] proposed that adding diet counseling and group session

Table 4.3 Summary of intervention impact on muscle mass

Study	Intervention group	Outcome and method	Impact of intervention	
			Post-intervention	Follow-up
de Jong et al. [26]	Nutrition: 58 Exercise: 55 Combination: 60 Control: 44	Lean body mass (kg); DXA	Exercise (0.2 ± 1.4 kg, $P<0.05$): significantly improved compared to control group (-0.5 ± 1.4 kg) Exercise ($n=75$) vs. no exercise ($n=68$): exercise ($+0.5 \pm 1.2$ kg, $P=0.02$), significantly improved compared to no exercise (-0.1 kg)	Not available data
Rydwik et al. [27]	Exercise + nutrition: 25 Nutrition: 25 Exercise: 23 Control: 23	FFM (kg) = (weight−fat mass) (fat mass = four skin folds using prediction equations)	NS	Within-group comparison: Exercise = -0.9 kg (95% CI = -1.7 to -0.2, $P<0.05$)
Kenny et al. [25]	Aerobics + placebo: 25 Aerobics + DHEA: 24 Yoga + placebo: 25 Yoga + DHEA: 25	Total and regional lean tissue mass (kg); DXA	Appendicular skeletal muscle mass: NS Lean mass: exercise + DHEA ($n=43$, 39.6 ± 6.1 kg), exercise + placebo ($n = 44$, 38.1 ± 5.2 kg), significant differences between groups ($P = 0.048$)	Not available data
Tieland et al. [24]	Exercise + protein: 31 Exercise + placebo: 31	Lean mass (kg); DXA	Treatment × time interactions; Lean mass: exercise + protein (47.2–48.5 kg), exercise + placebo (45.7–45.4 kg), $P = 0.006$ Appendicular lean mass: exercise + protein (20.1–21.0 kg), exercise + placebo (19.3–19.1 kg), $P < 0.001$	Not available data

(continued)

Table 4.3 (continued)

Study	Intervention group	Outcome and method	Impact of intervention	
			Post-intervention	Follow-up
Chan et al. [28]	Exercise + nutrition + PST: 28 Exercise + nutrition: 27 PST: 29 Control: 33	FFM (kg); BIA	Not available data	FFM: exercise (-0.46 ± 1.36 kg, $P < 0.05$), Non-exercise (-0.62 ± 1.84 kg, $P < 0.001$)
Kim et al. [29]	Exercise + nutrition: 33 Exercise + placebo: 33 Nutrition: 32 Placebo: 33	Appendicular skeletal (AS) and leg muscle mass (kg); DXA	Appendicular skeletal muscle mass: NS Leg muscle mass: Exercise + nutrition 2.4% (95% CI = 1.3–3.5)	Within-group comparison: AS mass: NS Leg muscle mass: Exercise + nutrition 3.2% (95% CI = 1.1–5.4), Exercise + placebo 3.2% (95% CI = 1.2–5.3)
Tarazona-Santabalbina et al. [30]	Exercise: 51 Control: 49	Lean mass (kg); BIA	NS	Not available data

Note: *DXA* dual X-ray absorptiometry, *FFM* fat-free mass, *BIA* bioelectrical impedance analysis, *PST* problem-solving therapy, *DHEA* dehydroepiandrosterone, *NS* not significant, *CI* confidence interval

education to physical training did not increase FFM post-intervention. Chan et al. [28] showed FFM declines in the exercise group (-0.46 ± 1.36 kg, $P < 0.05$) less than the non-exercise group (-0.62 ± 1.84 kg, $P < 0.01$)). Kim et al. [29] reported that leg muscle mass significantly increased in the exercise + nutrition group post-intervention, but post follow-up increases were also seen in the exercise + nutrition group as well as the exercise + placebo groups. Furthermore, Tarazona-Santabalbina et al. [30] found that adding exercise to nutritional advice and vitamin and mineral supplementation intervention did not significantly improve lean mass.

4.4.2.2 Change in Muscle Strength (Weakness)

Muscle strength was examined in many studies and in many ways: combining exercise and MFGM [29], exercise and BCAA [31], exercise and enriched foods [32], exercise and protein [24], exercise and cooking practice [33], exercise and diet counseling [27], exercise + nutritional supplementation + cognitive training [34], exercise and DHEA [25], and exercise and growth hormone [35] (Table 4.4). Among them, three studies showed treatment×time interaction.

Ng et al. [34] found in exercise + nutrition + cognitive, exercise alone, and cognitive alone showed significantly improved knee strength both at 6 months (cognitive = 2.18 kg, 95% CI = 1.08; 3.27; exercise = 2.75 kg, 95% CI = 1.66; 3.83; exercise + nutrition + cognitive = 2.67 kg, 95% CI = 1.58; 3.76) and at 12-month fol-

Table 4.4 Summary of intervention on muscle strength

Study	Intervention group	Outcome	Impact of intervention	
			Post-intervention	Follow-up
Chin A Paw et al. [32]	Exercise + enriched foods: 42 Exercise: 39 Enriched foods: 39 Control: 37	Upper (grip strength) Lower (quadriceps strength)	NS	Not available data
Hennessey et al. [35]	Exercise + growth hormone: 8 Growth hormone: 7 Exercise: 8 Control: 8	Lower (knee extension)	Exercise + growth hormone (+55.6%, $P = 0.0004$), exercise (+47.8%, $P = 0.0005$) significantly improved compared to baseline	Not available data
Rydwik et al. [27]	Exercise + nutrition: 25 Nutrition: 25 Exercise: 23 Control: 23	Upper (dips, Pulldown) Lower (leg press)	Within-group comparison Dips: exercise + nutrition (1.7 kg, 95% CI = 0.04; 3.4) and exercise (1.8 kg, 95% CI = 0.8; 2.8) change significantly improved Pulldown: exercise (3.4 kg, 95% CI = 0.9; 5.8) change significantly improved Leg press: exercise + nutrition (9 kg, 95% CI = 1.8; 16.2) and exercise (11.9 kg, 95% CI = 6.3; 17.5): change significantly improved	Within-group comparison Dips: NS Pulldown: exercise (2.7 kg, 95% CI = 0.9; 4.6) change significantly improved
Kenny et al. [25]	Aerobics + placebo: 25 Aerobics + DHEA: 24 Yoga + placebo: 25 Yoga + DHEA: 25	Upper (grip strength) Lower (leg press)	Grip strength: NS Leg press: treatment × time interactions ($P=0.015$) Exercise + DHEA (459 ± 121 N to 484±147 N, $P <0.05$) significantly improved compared to Exercise + placebo (477 ± 186 to 447±128 N, $P <0.05$)	Not available data
Tieland et al. [24]	Exercise + protein: 31 Exercise + placebo: 31	Upper (grip strength) Lower (leg press, leg extension)	NS	Not available data

(continued)

Table 4.4 (continued)

Study	Intervention group	Outcome	Impact of intervention	
			Post-intervention	Follow-up
Kim et al. [29]	Exercise + nutrition: 33 Exercise + placebo: 33 Nutrition: 32 Placebo: 33	Upper (grip strength) Lower (knee extension)	NS	NS
Kwon et al. [33]	Exercise: 28 Exercise + nutrition: 30 Control: 31	Upper (grip strength)	Within-group comparison Exercise + nutrition: NS Exercise (2.3 ± 3.1 kg, $P <0.05$) significantly improved compared to baseline	Within-group comparison Exercise (-0.3 ± 2.2 kg): NS Exercise+ nutrition (-2.1 ± 5.0 kg, $P <0.05$) significantly declined compared to post-intervention
Ng et al. [34]	Nutrition: 49 Cognitive training: 50 Exercise: 48 Combination: 49 Control: 50	Lower (knee extension)	Treatment × time interactions ($P = 0.009$) Within-group comparison: Significantly improved change compared between baseline and 6 months (cognitive = 2.18 kg, 95% CI = 1.08; 3.27), (exercise = 2.75 kg, 95% CI = 1.66; 3.83), (combination = 2.67 kg, 95% CI = 1.58; 3.76)	Treatment × time interactions ($P = 0.009$) Within-group comparison: Significantly improved change compared between baseline and 12 months (cognitive = 1.98 kg, 95% CI = 0.87; 3.09), (exercise = 1.41 kg, 95% CI = 0.31; 2.51), (combination = 2.35 kg, 95% CI = 1.25; 3.44)
Ikeda et al. [31]	Exercise + BCAA: 27 Control: 25	Upper (grip strength, rowing) Lower (leg press, hip abduction, knee extension)	Between group comparison Grip strength and rowing: NS Leg press: exercise + BCAA (13.9 ± 36.0%) significantly improved ($P = 0.032$) compared to control (2.7 ± 12.5%) Knee extension: exercise + BCAA (9.5 ± 26.3%) significantly improved ($P = 0.008$) compared to control ($-0.8 \pm 18.2\%$). NS for hip abduction	Not available data

Notes: *DHEA* dehydroepiandrosterone, *NS* not significant, *CI* confidence interval, *BCAA* branched-chain amino acids low-up (cognitive = 1.98 kg, 95% CI =0.87; 3.09; exercise = 1.41 kg, 95% CI =0.31; 2.51; exercise + nutrition + cognitive = 2.35 kg, 95% CI =1.25; 3.44) compared to the nutrition-alone and control group. Kenny et al. [25] found that adding a dehydroepian-drosterone (DHEA) supplementation (50 mg/day) to yoga or chair aerobics significantly improved leg press in exercise + DHEA (459 ± 121 N to 484 ± 147 N, $P < 0.05$) compared to exercise + placebo (477 ± 186 to 447 ± 128 N, $P < 0.05$) but not grip strength. Also, Ikeda et al. [31] found that adding the 6 g amino acid supplement to a strength, balance, and aerobic exercise intervention significantly improved leg press strength (13.9 ± 36.0%, $P = 0.032$) and knee extension strength (9.5 ± 26.3%, $P = 0.008$), but not for hip abduction strength, grip strength, and rowing. While interactions were not observed in these three studies, significant within-group improvements were reported. Rydwik et al. [27] found significantly improved leg press in both exercise + dietary counseling and exercise-alone groups (exercise + dietary counseling = 9.0 kg, 95% CI = 1.8–16.2; exercise = 11.9 kg, 95% CI = 6.3–17.5) and dips (exercise + dietary counseling = 1.7 kg, 95% CI = 0.04–3.4; exercise = 1.8 kg, 95% CI = 0.8–2.8) compared to baseline, but not significant at follow-up. Kwon et al. [33] found in the exercise alone group a significantly increased grip strength (2.3 ± 3.1 kg, $P < 0.05$), but no post-intervention significant increase were seen in the exercise + cooking class group. At 6-month follow-up, they found significantly declined grip strength in the exercise + cooking class group (−2.1 ± 5.0 kg, $P < 0.05$) compared to the exercise and control group. Hennessey et al. [35] found in exercise + growth hormone (+55.6%, $P = 0.0004$) and exercise alone (+47.8%, $P = 0.0005$) groups a significantly increased right knee extension strength at post-intervention.Some studies found no significant differences between baseline and post-intervention or follow-up: there was no significant effect in adding a milk fat globule membrane (MFGM) [29] or 15 g protein supplementation [24] to an exercise intervention. Chin A Paw et al. [32] found no significantly improved grip strength and quadriceps strength by an exercise or exercise combined with vitamin and mineral supplementation intervention compared to no exercise or nutritional alone intervention.

4.4.2.3 Change in Exhaustion

Three studies examined the effect of an intervention on exhaustion. Adding an exercise intervention to a MFGM supplementation or not and MFGM alone significantly improved exhaustion at follow-up ($P = 0.007$) [29]. However, two studies found no significant effect on exhaustion of adding dietary advices and PST to exercise [28] and multifactorial exercise intervention [36], respectively.

4.4.2.4 Change in Gait Speed

Eight studies measured gait speed (Table 4.5), and three found treatment×time interactions. Kim et al. [29] found that adding an exercise intervention to MFGM supplementation significantly improved usual walking speed (exercise + MFGM = 14.7 ± 4.1%,

Table 4.5 Summary of intervention on gait speed

Study	Intervention group	Outcome	Impact of intervention	
			Post-intervention	Follow-up
Chin A Paw et al. [32]	Exercise + enriched foods: 42 Exercise: 39 Enriched foods: 39 Control: 37	Usual walking speed	Exercise ($n = 81$, 0.06 ± 0.1 meter/ seconds): significantly improved compared to no exercise ($n = 76$, 0.0 ± 0.04 meter/ seconds, $P < 0.004$)	Not available data
Rydwik et al. [27]	Exercise + nutrition: 25 Nutrition: 25 Exercise: 23 Control: 23	Maximal walking speed	NS	NS
Kenny et al. [25]	Aerobics + placebo: 25 Aerobics + DHEA: 24 Yoga + placebo: 25 Yoga + DHEA: 25	Walking speed	NS	NS
Tieland et al. [24]	Exercise + protein: 31 Exercise + placebo: 31	Gait speed	NS	Not available data
Cameron et al. [36]	Multifactorial: 120 Control: 121	Gait speed	NS	Between group difference: intervention (-0.049 ± 0.183 meter/ seconds) significantly improved compared to control (0.019 ± 0.230 meter/ seconds), ($P = 0.02$)
Kwon et al. [33]	Exercise: 28 Exercise + nutrition: 30 Control: 31	Usual walking speed	NS	NS
Kim et al. [29]	Exercise + nutrition: 33 Exercise + placebo: 33 Nutrition: 32 Placebo: 33	Usual walking speed	Treatment × time interactions ($P = 0.005$) Exercise + nutrition ($14.7 \pm 4.1\%$, 95% CI = 6.4; 23.1) change significantly improved compared to nutrition ($2.1 \pm 1.9\%$, 95% CI = -1.8; 5.9) or placebo ($3.6 \pm 2.7\%$, 95% CI = -1.9; 9.1)	NS
Ng et al. [34]	Nutrition: 49 Cognitive training: 50 Exercise: 48 Combination: 49 Control: 50	Maximal walking speed	Treatment × time interactions: NS Within-group comparison: exercise (-1.29 m, 95% CI = -1.72; -0.85) significantly improved ($P<0.05$)	Treatment × time interactions: NS Within-group comparison, Exercise: 6 months (-1.10 m, 95% CI = -1.53; -0.67) and 12 months (-1.14 m, 95% CI = -1.58; -0.70) significantly improved ($P<0.05$)

Note: *DHEA* dehydroepiandrosterone, *NS* not significant, *CI* confidence interval

95% CI =6.4; 23.1) compared to MFGM (2.1 ± 1.9%, 95% CI = −1.8; 5.9) or placebo (3.6 ± 2.7%, 95% CI = −1.9; 9.1) ($P = 0.026$). Cameron et al. [36] did not find significant changes between baseline and 3 months. Baseline and 12-month comparisons showed that multifactorial interdisciplinary intervention (−0.049 ± 0.183 meter/seconds) significantly improved compared to control (0.019 ± 0.230 meter/seconds) ($P = 0.02$). Chin A Paw et al. [32] showed no significant changes when comparing four interventions. A two-factorial analysis between exercise ($n = 81$, exercise alone and exercise + enriched foods) and non-exercise ($n = 76$, enriched foods and control) revealed significant improvements in usual walking speed for exercise intervention (0.06 ± 0.1 meter/seconds) compared to no exercise (0.0 ± 0.04 meter/seconds, $P < 0.004$). In one study, although treatment × time interactions were not observed, within-group comparisons found significant changes. Ng et al. [34] found that while 3 months of strength and balance training significantly improved maximal walking speed (−1.29 m, 95% CI = −1.72; −0.85), there were no significant improvements in nutrition, cognitive, combined, and control groups. Further, only the exercise group significantly improved at the 6-month (−1.10 m, 95% CI = −1.53; −0.67) and 12-month (−1.14 m, 95% CI = −1.58; −0.70) follow-up. Adding nutritional advice and cooking class or protein supplementation to an exercise intervention showed no significant effect on gait speed, compared to exercise intervention alone [27, 33]. Also, adding a DHEA supplementation to yoga or chair aerobics exercise intervention showed no significant effect for walking speed [25].

4.4.2.5 Change in Physical Activity Level

Eight studies examined the effect interventions on physical activity level (Table 4.6). Adding an exercise intervention to nutritional advice and vitamin and mineral supplementation significantly improved low physical activity in exercise (485.6 ± 98.1) compared to the control (265.8 ± 46.1), $P < 0.001$ [30]. Low physical activity was also significantly improved by exercise alone or exercise combined with nutrition post-intervention and at 6-month follow-up. In addition, this increase remained in the exercise group compared to nutrition or control group [37]. Another three studies found no significant effect on physical activity level at post-intervention, but significantly increased physical activity level by a multifactorial exercise [36], exercise + MFGM [29], and nutrition-alone [34] intervention compared to the control group or baseline at follow-up. However, three studies found no significant effect on physical activity level of adding a hormone supplementation to exercise [25], adding dietary advices and PST to exercise [28], and adding a protein supplementation to exercise intervention Ikeda et al. [31], respectively.

Change in Frailty Status

Previous studies assessed the impact of a multi-domain intervention including exercise, nutritional supplementation, hormone supplementation, diet advice, cooking class, social support, and cognitive training on frailty status such as frail, prefrail, and robust (Table 4.7). Post-intervention, some studies found a significantly

Table 4.6 Summary of intervention on physical activity

Study	Intervention group	Outcome	Impact of intervention Post-intervention	Follow-up
Rydwik et al. [37]	Exercise + nutrition: 25 Nutrition: 25 Exercise: 23 Control: 23	Classification of physical activity	Exercise and exercise + nutrition groups significantly increased compared to control group	Exercise group significantly improved compared to nutrition and control groups
Kenny et al. [25]	Aerobics + placebo: 25 Aerobics + DHEA: 24 Yoga + placebo: 25 Yoga + DHEA: 25	Physical activity scale (kcal/wk)	NS	Not available data
Chan et al. [28]	Exercise + nutrition + PST: 28 Exercise + nutrition: 27 PST: 29 Control: 33	International physical activity questionnaire short form Weekly energy expenditure	NS	NS
Cameron et al. [36]	Multifactorial: 120 Control: 121	Energy expenditure	NS	Low physical activity significantly improved in intervention (63%) compared to control (76%), and the between-group difference was 12.9% (95% CI = −25.2; −0.6, P = 0.04)
Kim et al. [29]	Exercise + nutrition: 33 Exercise + placebo: 33 Nutrition: 32 Placebo: 33	Three or more of the following activity: Regular walking, <once a week Regular exercise, no Hobbies activity, no Volunteering activity, no	NS	Low physical activity significantly improved in exercise + MFGM (36.4%) compared to exercise + placebo (9.1%), MFGM (9.4%), and control (9.1%) groups (P = 0.004)

Ng et al. [34]	Nutrition: 49 Cognitive training: 50 Exercise: 48 Combination: 49 Control: 50	31-item longitudinal aging physical activity questionnaire (self-reported)	NS	6 months: nutrition (mean change = 96.2, 95%CI = 57.8; 134.7) significantly improved compared to baseline 12 months: nutrition (mean change = 110.1, 95%CI = 71.9; 148.2) significantly improved compared to baseline
Ikeda et al. [31]	Exercise + BCAA: 27 Control: 25	Frenchay activities index	NS	Not available data
Tarazona-Santabalbina et al. [30]	Exercise: 51 Control: 49	Physical activity energetic expenditure	Exercise (485.6 ± 98.1) significantly improved compared to control group (265.8 ± 46.1), $P < 0.001$.	Not available data

Notes: *NS* not significant, *BCAA* branched-chain amino acids, *CI* confidence interval, *MFGM* milk fat globule membrane

Table 4.7 Summary of intervention impact on frailty status

Study	Study participants	Intervention group	Outcome	Impact of intervention Post-intervention	Follow-up
Cameron et al. [36]	Frail	Exercise (Multifactorial): 120 Control: 121	Frailty and mobility	NS	Frailty: Exercise (62%), Control (76%), % difference=14.7%, $P = 0.02$
Kim et al. [29]	Frail	Exercise + nutrition: 33 Exercise + placebo: 33 Nutrition: 32 Placebo: 33	Reversal rate of frailty status	Reversal rates: significantly higher in exercise + nutrition (57.6%) than nutrition (28.1%) or placebo (30.3%) groups, $P = 0.032$	Reversal rates: significantly higher in exercise + nutrition (45.5%) and exercise + placebo (39.4%) than placebo (15.2%) group, $P = 0.035$
Chan et al. [28]	Prefrail and frail	Exercise + nutrition + PST: 28 Exercise + nutrition: 27 PST: 29 Control: 33	Improvement of CHS criteria by at least one category	Improvement of one category: significantly higher in exercise + nutrition (45%) than non-exercise + non-nutrition (27%) group, $P = 0.008$	NS
Ng et al. [34]	Prefrail and frail	Nutrition: 49 Cognitive training: 50 Exercise: 48 Combination: 49 Control: 50	Reduction of frailty	Not available data	Frailty reduction: significantly higher in nutrition (35.6%), cognitive (35.6%), exercise (41.3%), and combination (47.8%) than control (15.2%) group, $P<0.01$
Luger et al. [38]	Prefrail and frail	Exercise + nutrition: 39 Social support: 41	Change of frailty prevalence	NS	Not available data

Note: *NS* not significant, *PST* problem-solving therapy, *CHS* cardiovascular health study improved frailty status or frailty criteria in the multi-domain intervention groups such as exercise + MFGM [29], exercise + nutrition + cognitive training [34], exercise + diet advices + PST [28], and exercise + diet advices + protein intake [37] compared to single-domain such as exercise-alone or nutrition-alone intervention groups or control group. The primary outcomes in two studies were frailty status reversal [29, 36], prefrail or frailty improvement in three studies [28, 34, 38], and, in one study, changes in frailty criteria [30].

Post-intervention results in one study showed significantly higher reversal rates in exercise + MFGM (57.6%) than MFGM alone (28.1%) or placebo (30.3%) groups ($P = 0.032$). Also, at 4-month follow-up, larger significant improvements were maintained in groups with an exercise intervention irrespective of their additional nutritional supplementation (exercise + MFGM = 45.5%, exercise + placebo = 39.4%) compared to placebo (15.2%) for frailty status ($P = 0.035$) [29]. In another study [36], participants of the multifactorial interdisciplinary intervention did not reverse frailty status at post-intervention. At 12-month follow-up, there was a lower prevalence of frailty in the intervention group (62%) compared with the control group (76%); the between-group difference in frailty was 14.7% (95% CI = 2.4–27.0, $P = 0.02$).

Chan et al. [28] found a significantly higher improvement of one category in exercise + diet advices group (45%) compared with non-exercise and nutrition group (27%) at post-intervention. But, participants of the exercise + diet advices + PST intervention did not maintain its significant larger improvement of frailty status at 6-month and 12-month follow-up compared to control or a PST intervention. Ng et al. [34], at 12-month follow-up, showed a significantly improved frailty status in nutrition (35.6%), cognitive (35.6%), exercise (41.3%), and combination (47.8%) than control (15.2%) group ($P < 0.01$).

At post-intervention, one study observed significantly lowering score assessed by Fried frailty criteria and Edmonton frailty scale in intervention groups compared to control group [30]. However, one study found no significant difference on frailty status between an exercise + nutrition (−17%) and a social support (−16%) intervention [38].

Overall, multi-domain interventions showed significantly larger improved frailty status and score compared to single-domain or control interventions.

4.5 Conclusion

Frailty is highly prevalent and associated with substantial morbidity and poor health outcomes. Various factors cause frailty in elderly people including chronic disease, lack of physical activity, malnutrition, and aging itself, some of which are unpreventable. Exercise and nutritional supplementation are among the beneficial treatments promoting healthy and independent lifestyles in the elderly. Evidence reveals that exercise targeted at reducing risk factors is an effective strategy for preventing and/or treating frailty in elderly people. Progressive and moderate-intensity exercise alone or combined with nutritional and hormone supplementation should be encouraged among elderly people to minimize the degenerative physical, psychological, social, and cognitive function that occurs with aging.

References

1. Woods NF, LaCroix AZ, Gray SL, et al. Frailty: Emergence and consequences in women aged 65 and older in the women's health initiative observational study. J Am Geriatr Soc. 2005;53:1321–30.
2. Vermeiren S, Vella-Azzopardi R, Beckwee D, et al. Frailty and the prediction of negative health outcomes: aA meta-analysis. J Am Med Dir Assoc. 2016;17:1163.e1–1163.e17.
3. Fried LP, Tangen CM, Walston J, et al. Frailty in older adults: evidence for a phenotype. J Gerontol A Biol Sci Med Sci. 2001;56:M146–56.
4. Winograd CH, Gerety MB, Chung M, et al. Screening for frailty: Criteria and predictors of outcomes. J Am Geriatr Soc. 1991;39:778–84.
5. Speechley M, Tinetti M. Falls and injuries in frail and vigorous community elderly persons. J Am Geriatr Soc. 1991;39:46–52.
6. Rolfson DB, Majumdar SR, Tsuyuki RT, et al. Validity and reliability of the Edmonton frail scale. Age Ageing. 2006;35:526–9.
7. Bandeen-Roche K, Xue QL, Ferrucci L, et al. Phenotype of frailty: characterization in the women's health and aging studies. J Gerontol A Biol Sci Med Sci. 2006;61:262–6.
8. Satake S, Shimada H, Yamada M, et al. Prevalence of frailty among community-dwellers and outpatients in Japan as defined by the Japanese version of the Cardiovascular Health Study criteria. Geriatr Gerontol Int. 2017;17:2629–34. https://doi.org/10.1111/ggi.13129.
9. van Oostrom SH, van der ADL, Rietman ML, et al. A four-domain approach of frailty explored in the Doetinchem cohort study. BMC GeriatrBMC Geriatrics. 2017;17:196. https://doi.org/10.1186/s12877-017-0595-0.
10. Collard RM, Boter H, Schoevers RA, et al. Prevalence of frailty in community-dwelling older persons: a systematic review. J Am Geriatr Soc. 2012;60:1487–92.
11. Sirven N, Rapp T. The cost of frailty in France. Eur J Health Econ. 2017;18:243–53.
12. Walston J, Hadley EC, Ferrucci L, et al. Research agenda for frailty in older adults: toward a better understanding of physiology and etiology: summary from the American Geriatrics Society/National Institute on Aging Research Conference on Frailty in Older Adults. J Am Geriatr Soc. 2006;54:991–1001.
13. Xue QL, Bandeen-Roche K, Varadhan R, et al. Initial manifestations of frailty criteria and the development of frailty phenotype in the Women's Health and Aging Study II. J Gerontol A Biol Sci Med Sci. 2008;63:984–90.
14. Makizako H, Shimada H, Doi T, et al. Impact of physical frailty on disability in community-dwelling older adults: a prospective cohort study. BMJ Open. 2015;e0048462:5.
15. Dillon EL, Sheffield-Moore M, Paddon-Jones D, et al. Amino acid supplementation increases lean body mass, basal muscle protein synthesis, and insulin-like growth factor-I expression in older women. J Clin Endocrinol Metab. 2009;94:1630–7.
16. Fiatarone MA, O'Neill EF, Ryan ND, et al. Exercise training and nutritional supplementation for physical frailty in very elderly people. N Engl J Med. 1994;330:1769–75.
17. Liu CJ, Latham NK. Progressive resistance strength training for improving physical function in older adults. Cochrane Database Syst Rev. 2009;8:CD002759. https://doi.org/10.1002/14651858.CD002759.pub2.
18. Borst SE. Interventions for sarcopenia and muscle weakness in older people. Age Ageing. 2004;33:548–55.

19. Peterson MD, Sen A, Gordon PM. Influence of resistance exercise on lean body mass in aging adults: A meta-analysis. Med Sci Sports Exerc. 2011;43:249–58.
20. Taaffe DR. Sarcopenia – exercise as a treatment strategy. Aust Fam Physician. 2006;35:130–4.
21. Kim H, Suzuki T, Saito K, et al. Effects of exercise and amino acid supplementation on body composition and physical function in community-welling elderly Japanese sarcopenic women: A randomized controlled trial. J Am Geriatr Soc. 2012;60:16–23.
22. Dedeyne L, Deschodt M, Verschueren S, et al. Effects of multi-domain interventions in (pre) frail elderly on frailty, functional, and cognitive status: a systematic review. Clin Interv Aging. 2017;12:873–96.
23. Puts MTE, Toubasi S, Andrew MK, et al. Interventions to prevent or reduce the level of frailty in community-dwelling older adults: a scoping review of the literature and international policies. Age Ageing. 2017;46:383–92.
24. Tieland M, Dirks ML, van der Zwaluw N, et al. Protein supplementation increases muscle mass gain during prolonged resistance-type exercise training in frail elderly people: a randomized, double-blind, placebo-controlled trial. J Am Med Dir Assoc. 2012;13:713–9.
25. Kenny AM, Boxer RS, Kleppinger A, et al. Dehydroepiandrosterone combined with exercise improves muscle strength and physical function in frail older women. J Am Geriatr Soc. 2010;58:1707–14.
26. de Jong N, Chin A Paw MJM, de Groot LCPGM, et al. Dietary supplements and physical exercise affecting bone and body composition in frail elderly persons. Am J Public Health. 2000;90:947–54.
27. Rydwik E, Lammes E, Frandin K, et al. Effects of a physical and nutritional intervention program for frail elderly people over age 75. A randomized controlled pilot treatment trial. Aging Clin Exp Res. 2008;20:159–70.
28. Chan DC, Tsou HH, Yang RS, et al. A pilot randomized controlled trial to improve geriatric frailty. BMC Geriatr. 2012;12:58. https://doi.org/10.1186/1471-2318-12-58.
29. Kim H, Suzuki T, Kim M, et al. Effects of exercise and milk fat globule membrane (MFGM) supplementation on body composition, physical function, and hematological parameters in community-dwelling frail Japanese women: a randomized double blind, placebo-controlled, follow-up trial. PLoS One. 2015;10:e0116256.
30. Tarazona-Santabalbina F, Gomez-Cabrera M, Perez-Ros P, et al. A multicomponent exercise intervention that reverses frailty and improves cognition, emotion, and social networking in the community-dwelling frail elderly: a randomized clinical trial. J Am Med Dir Assoc. 2016;17:426–33.
31. Ikeda T, Aizawa J, Nagasawa H, et al. Effects and feasibility of exercise therapy combined with branched-chain amino acid supplementation on muscle strengthening in frail and pre-frail elderly people requiring long-term care: a crossover trial. Appl Physiol Nutr Metab. 2016;41:438–45.
32. Chin A Paw MJM, de Jong N, Schouten EG, et al. Physical exercise and/or enriched foods for functional improvement in frail, independently living elderly: a randomized controlled trial. Arch Phys Med Rehabil. 2001;82:811–7.
33. Kwon J, Yoshida Y, Yoshida H, et al. Effects of a combined physical training and nutrition intervention on physical performance and health-related quality of life in prefrail older women living in the community: a randomized controlled trial. J Am Med Dir Assoc. 2015;16:261–8.
34. Ng TP, Feng L, Zin Nyunt MS, et al. Nutritional, physical, cognitive, and combination interventions and frailty reversal among older adults: a randomized controlled trial. Am J Med. 2015;128:1225.e1–36.e1.
35. Hennessey JV, Chromiak JA, Ventura SD, et al. Growth hormone administration and exercise effects on muscle fiber type and diameter in moderately frail older people. J Am Geriatr Soc. 2001;49:852–8.

36. Cameron ID, Fairhall N, Langron C, et al. A multifactorial interdisciplinary intervention reduces frailty in older people: randomized trial. BMC Med. 2013;11:65. https://doi.org/10.1186/1741-7015-11-65.
37. Rydwik E, Frandin K, Akner G. Effects of a physical training and nutritional intervention program in frail elderly people regarding habitual physical activity level and activities of daily living – a randomized controlled pilot study. Arch Gerontol Geriatr. 2010;51:283–9.
38. Luger E, Dorner TE, Haider S, et al. Effects of a home-based and volunteer-administered physical training, nutritional, and social support program on malnutrition and frailty in older persons: a randomized controlled trial. J Am Med Dir AssocJ Am Med Dir Assoc. 2016;17:671. e9–671.e16.

Chapter 5
Epidemiology of the Locomotive Organ Diseases

Noriko Yoshimura, Kozo Nakamura, and Sakae Tanaka

Abstract Although locomotive organ disorders are major causes of disability and require support, little information is available regarding their epidemiology. In this chapter, epidemiological indices such as prevalence of locomotive organ diseases including knee osteoarthritis, lumbar spondylosis, hip osteoarthritis, osteoporosis, and sarcopenia and their coexistence were clarified using results of the research on osteoarthritis/osteoporosis against disability (ROAD) study, in addition, mutual effect of osteoarthritis, osteoporosis, and sarcopenia.

The prevalence of knee pain, lumbar pain, and their coexistence using the survey results of the longitudinal cohorts of motor system organ (LOCOMO) study was also clarified. It was found that the presence of knee pain affected lumbar pain and vice versa.

Finally, data from the third survey (7-year follow-up) of the ROAD study were used to estimate the prevalence of the locomotive syndrome using tests proposed by the Japanese Orthopaedic Association for assessing the risk of developing locomotive syndrome. Subsequently, the age-sex prevalence of stage 1 and stage 2 locomotive syndrome was estimated at 69.8% and 25.1%, respectively.

Keywords Osteoarthritis · Osteoporosis · Sarcopenia · Knee pain · Lumbar pain · Locomotive syndrome at stages 1 and 2 · Population-based cohort study

N. Yoshimura (✉)
Department of Preventive Medicine for Locomotive Organ Disorders, 22nd Century Medical and Research Center, The University of Tokyo, Tokyo, Japan
e-mail: yoshimuran-ort@h.u-tokyo.ac.jp

K. Nakamura
National Rehabilitation Center for Persons with Disabilities, Saitama, Japan

S. Tanaka
Department of Orthopaedic Surgery, Sensory and Motor System Medicine, Graduate School of Medicine, The University of Tokyo, Tokyo, Japan

© Springer Nature Singapore Pte Ltd. 2019
M. Washio, C. Kiyohara (eds.), *Health Issues and Care System for the Elderly*,
Current Topics in Environmental Health and Preventive Medicine,
https://doi.org/10.1007/978-981-13-1762-0_5

5.1 Introduction

According to the recent National Livelihood Survey undertaken by the Ministry of Health, Labour, and Welfare in Japan, the leading cause of disability requiring support or long-term care is dementia, followed by cardiovascular disease and senility [1]. Osteoporotic fractures and falls are ranked fourth, while osteoarthritis (OA) is ranked fifth; their combined contribution is much higher than that of dementia. Besides, musculoskeletal diseases can affect joint pain, mobile function, activities of daily living, and quality of life. Given the increasing proportion of elderly individuals in the Japanese population, a comprehensive and evidence-based prevention strategy for musculoskeletal diseases is urgently required.

The Japanese Orthopaedic Association (JOA) proposed the term 'locomotive syndrome' to designate a condition requiring nursing care or the risk of developing such a condition, following a decline in mobility resulting from one or more disorders of the locomotive organs, which include the bones, joints, muscles, and nerves [2]. The weakness of locomotive organs causes difficulty in mobility, which is defined as the ability to stand, walk, run, climb stairs, and perform other physical functions essential to daily life. In addition, the JOA proposed the following three tests as candidate indices to assess the risk of developing the locomotive syndrome in 2013: the two-step test, stand-up test, and 25-question geriatric locomotive function scale (GLFS) [3]. Furthermore, the JOA determined the clinical decision limits of these indices for assessing the risk of locomotive syndrome [4].

To prevent onset of locomotive organ diseases and progression to disability, it is important to clarify epidemiological indices such as prevalence, coexistence, or mutual association of locomotive organ diseases. However, little information is available regarding the epidemiology of the locomotive syndrome and/or locomotive organ diseases, because only a few prospective, longitudinal studies have been conducted in this area, especially for musculoskeletal diseases. The research on osteoarthritis/osteoporosis against disability (ROAD) study, which started in 2005, is a prospective cohort study that aims to elucidate the environmental and genetic background for bone and joint diseases. It was designed to examine the extent to which risk factors for these diseases are related to clinical features, laboratory and radiographic findings, bone mass and geometry, lifestyle, nutritional factors, anthropometric and neuromuscular measures, and fall propensity [5, 6]. The 3-year follow-up (second survey) of the ROAD study was conducted with residents of the same communities in 2008–2010, the 7-year follow-up (third survey) was in 2012–2013, and the 10-year follow-up (fourth survey) has completed at the end of 2016.

In this chapter, epidemiological indices such as the prevalence and coexistence of locomotive organ diseases including OA of the knee, lumbar spine, and hip, osteoporosis (OP) diagnosed at lumbar spine L2–4 and femoral neck, and sarcopenia (SP) are clarified. Further, mutual associations among locomotive organ diseases, such as KOA, LS, and OP, using baseline and 3-year follow-up data from the ROAD study are described. Next, the prevalences of knee and lumbar pain, using the results of the longitudinal cohorts of motor system organ (LOCOMO) study, details of which are described later, are noted. Finally, using information collected in the third survey (7-year follow-up) of the ROAD study, the prevalence of the locomotive syndrome, using tests proposed by the JOA for assessing the risk of developing it, is shown.

5.2 Prevalence of Locomotive Organ Diseases

In this section, the results of the above-mentioned ROAD study are cited. Recruitment methods for this study have been described in detail elsewhere [5, 6]. The baseline database includes clinical and genetic information of 3040 inhabitants (1061 men and 1979 women) aged 23–95 years who were recruited from the resident registries of three Japanese communities. All participants provided written informed consent, and the study was conducted with approval from the ethics committees of the participating institutions.

5.2.1 Prevalence of Knee Osteoarthritis (KOA), Lumbar Spondylosis (LS), and Hip Osteoarthritis (OA), and Their Coexistence

Plain radiographs with anteroposterior and lateral views of the lumbar spine and an anteroposterior view of the bilateral knees and hips with weight-bearing and foot-map positioning were obtained. The severity of radiographic OA was determined according to the Kellgren-Lawrence (KL) scale [7]. Radiographs of the knees, hips, and vertebrae were examined by a single, experienced orthopaedic surgeon who was unaware of the participants' clinical status. If at least one joint was graded as KL2 or higher, the participant was diagnosed with radiographic OA.

Figure 5.1 shows the age-sex distribution for the prevalence of radiographic KOA as determined by a KL grade ≥ 2 [5]. In the overall population, prevalence of radiographic KOA was 54.6% (42.0% in men and 61.5% in women), and it was significantly higher in women than in men ($P < 0.001$). The prevalence of radiographic KOA tended to be higher with age in both sexes.

Figure 5.1 also shows the prevalence of radiographic LS as determined by a KL grade ≥ 2 [5]. The prevalence of radiographic LS was 70.2% (80.6% in men and 64.6% in women), and tended to be higher with age in both sexes. Unlike radiographic KOA, the prevalence was significantly higher in men than in women ($P < 0.001$).

Figure 5.2 shows the prevalence of radiographic hip OA as determined by a KL grade ≥ 2 [8]. Overall, the prevalence 15.7% (18.2% in men and 14.3% in women), but unlike radiographic KOA and LS, the prevalence of hip OA tended not to be higher with age. The prevalence was significantly higher in men than in women ($P < 0.05$).

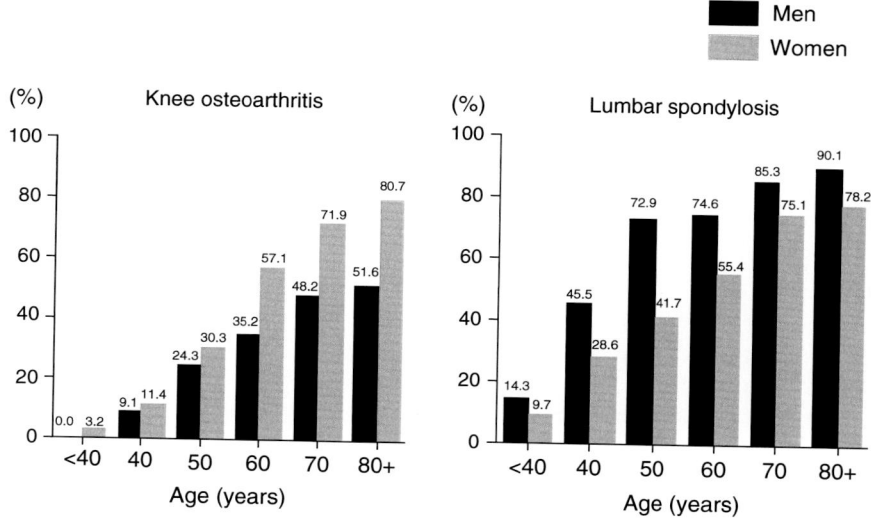

Fig. 5.1 Prevalence (%) of knee osteoarthritis and lumbar spondylosis with a Kellgren-Lawrence grade ≥2. Yoshimura N, et al. J Bone Miner Metab 27: 620–628, 2009

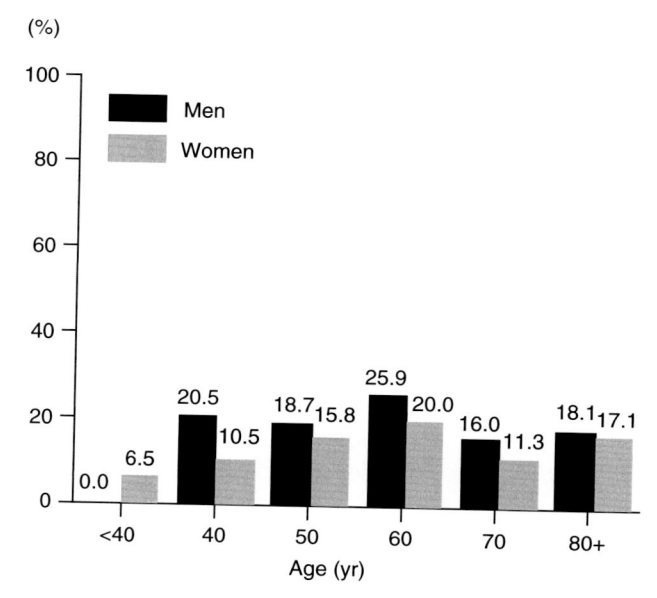

Fig. 5.2 Prevalence (%) of hip osteoarthritis with a Kellgren-Lawrence grade ≥2. Iidaka T, et al. Osteoarthritis Cartilage 24: 117–123, 2016

Fig. 5.3 Coexistence (%) of knee osteoarthritis, lumbar spondylosis, and hip osteoarthritis. Yoshimura N, et al. Mod Rheumatol 27: 1–7, 2017

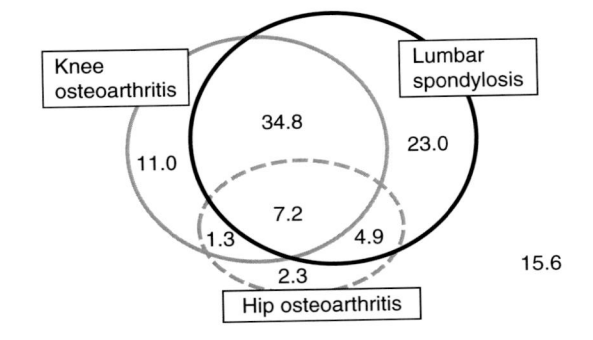

The present study clarified the prevalence of radiographic KOA, LS, and hip OA according to age and sex in some Japanese communities. If the ROAD study results are applied to the total age-sex distribution according to the 2005 Japanese census [9], 25,300,000 (8,600,000 men, 16,700,000 women), 37,900,000 (18,900,000 men, 19,000,000 women), and 12,000,000 (6,600,000 men and 5,400,000 women) people aged 40 years and older would be affected by radiographic KOA, LS, and hip OA, respectively, even though this estimation includes asymptomatic OA.

Figure 5.3 shows a Venn diagram representing the overlap of KOA, LS, and hip OA in the whole population. KOA and LS coexistence was most common and observed in 42.0% of the population. Coexistence of KOA, LS, and hip OA was observed in 7.2% of the population. KOA alone was present in 11.0%, LS in 23.0%, and hip OA in 2.3% of people, while 15.6% had none of these diseases [10].

5.2.2 Prevalence of OP and SP and Their Coexistence

For all 1690 of the 3040 baseline ROAD survey participants from mountainous and coastal areas, bone mineral density (BMD) was measured at the lumbar spine L2–4 and the proximal femur using dual-energy X-ray absorptiometry (DXA; Hologic Discovery, Hologic, Waltham, MA, USA). The same physician examined all participants to prevent observer variability. OP was defined by the Japanese Society for Bone and Mineral Research criteria [11]. A BMD of <0.708 g/cm^2 at the lumbar spine L2–4 in both men and women and a BMD of <0.604 g/cm^2 at the femoral neck in men and <0.551 g/cm^2 in women were all defined as OP.

Figure 5.4 reveals the prevalence of OP at the lumbar spine and femoral neck among residents of mountainous and coastal regions in the ROAD study. The prevalence of OP at the lumbar spine and femoral neck in women was six- and twofold significantly higher, respectively, than in men ($P < 0.001$). Considering the total age-sex distribution according to the Japanese census in 2005 [9], we can assume that 6,400,000 people (800,000 men, 5,600,000 women) aged 40 years and older

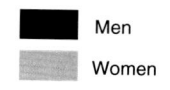

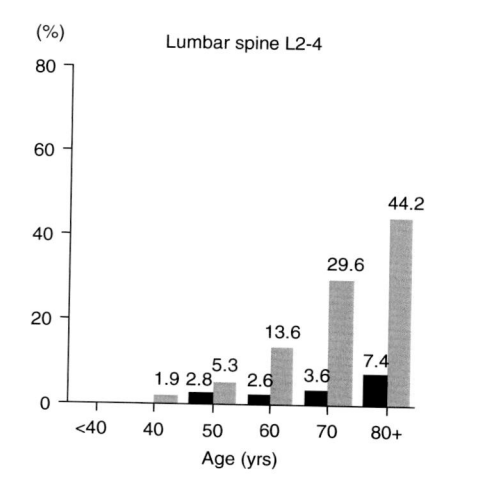

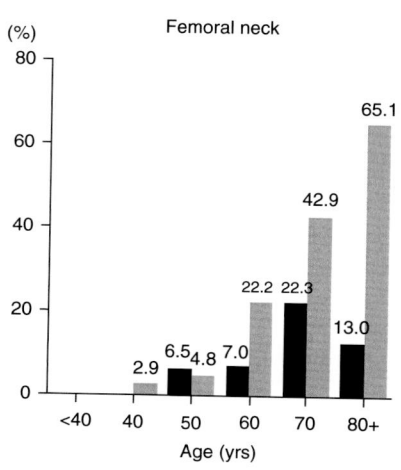

Fig. 5.4 Prevalence (%) of osteoporosis at the lumbar spine L2–4 and femoral neck. Yoshimura N, et al. J Bone Miner Metab 27: 620–628, 2009

had OP at the lumbar spine L2–4, while 10,700,000 (2,600,000 men, 8,100,000 women) of the same cohort had OP at the femoral neck.

The prevalence of the presence of OP either at the lumbar spine L2–4 or femoral neck in participants aged <40, 40–49, 50–59, 60–69, 70–79, and ≥80 years was 0.0%, 2.7%, 8.2%, 20.8%, 39.8%, and 54.4%, respectively (0.0%, 0.0%, 9.4%, 7.6%, 23.6%, and 16.7%, respectively, in men and 0.0%, 3.8%, 7.7%, 27.2%, 50.9%, and 74.0%, respectively, in women). Further, based on the total age-sex distributions according to the Japanese census in 2005 [9], 12,800,000 people (3,000,000 men, 9,800,000 women) aged 40 years and older were affected by OP at either the lumbar spine L2–4 or femoral neck.

In the elderly, SP is characterised by generalised loss of skeletal muscle mass and muscle strength and/or function, causing multiple adverse health outcomes. The Asian Working Group for Sarcopenia (AWGS) announced the appropriate diagnostic cut-off values for Asian populations in 2014 [12]. In the ROAD study, second and third surveys were performed to clarify SP prevalence and cumulative incidence using the AWGS criteria, determine the coexisting proportions of SP and OP, and evaluate whether there was a significant contribution of SP to subsequent OP development or vice versa in elderly Japanese subjects.

SP prevalences according to age group stratifications of 60–64, 65–69, 70–74, 75–79, and ≥80 years were 0.5%, 0.0%, 4.3%, 11.2%, and 27.0%, respectively (men, 1.5%, 0.0%, 4.7%, 11.5%, and 23.9%, for 60–64, 65–69, 70–74, 75–79, and

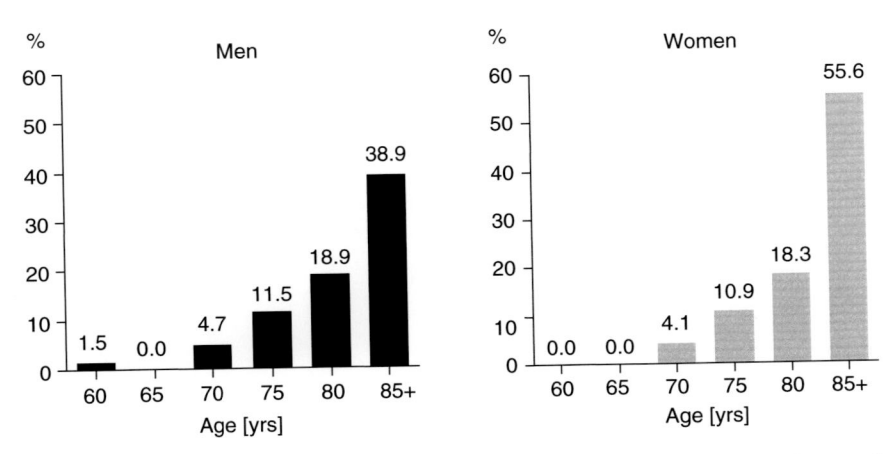

Fig. 5.5 Prevalence (%) of sarcopenia using the criteria of Asian Working Group for Sarcopenia. Yoshimura N, Osteoporos Int 28: 189–199, 2017

≥80 years, respectively; women, 0.0%, 0.0%, 4.1%, 10.9%, and 28.7%, for 60–64, 65–69, 70–74, 75–79, and ≥80 years, respectively). Above the age of 70 years, SP prevalence increased in an age-dependent manner, but there was no significant difference in prevalence according to sex (Fig. 5.5) [13].

In the population aged ≥60 years, SP and OP coexistence was observed in 4.7%, SP alone was present in 3.5%, OP alone was noted in 20.2%, and 71.7% had neither SP nor OP.

In men, the prevalence of coexisting SP and OP, SP alone, OP alone, and neither SP nor OP were 1.9%, 6.7%, 5.1%, and 86.4%, respectively, and in women, those were 6.2%, 1.8%, 28.0%, and 63.9%, respectively. The difference in distribution in prevalence between men and women was most significant for OP. That is, prevalence of the coexistence of SP and OP, and OP alone were significantly higher in women compared with men (p < 0.001) [13].

5.2.3 Mutual Associations Between Locomotive Organ Diseases, Such as KOA, LS, and OP

Of the 1690 baseline survey participants from mountainous and coastal regions of the ROAD study, 1384 (81.9%; 466 men, 918 women) completed all the examinations at the 3-year follow-up.

Figure 5.6 reveals the mutual associations among locomotive organ diseases, such as KOA, LS, and OP. The risk of the occurrence of OP at L2–4 was increased by the presence of OP at the femoral neck ($P = 0.008$), and the risk of the occurrence of OP at the femoral neck was increased by the presence of OP at L2–4 ($P = 0.047$)

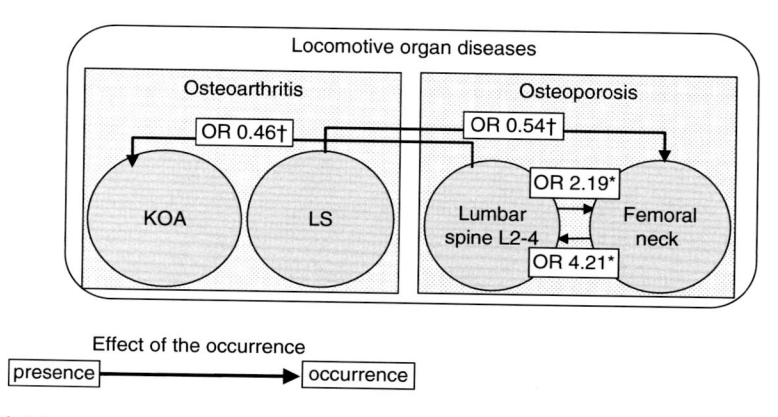

Fig. 5.6 Mutual associations among locomotive organ diseases, such as knee osteoarthritis, lumbar spondylosis, and osteoporosis. $^\dagger P < 0.1$, $^* P < 0.05$. Logistic regression analysis was performed after adjustment for age, gender, residing area, smoking habit, and drinking habit. *KOA* knee osteoarthritis, *LS* lumbar spondylosis. Yoshimura N, et al. Mod Rheumatol 25: 38–48, 2015

(Fig. 5.6) [14]. The presence of OP at lumbar L2–4 tended to decrease the risk of the occurrence of KOA, and the presence of LS tended to decrease the risk of the occurrence of OP at the femoral neck, although both of these associations were not statistically significant.

Regarding the mutual association between OP and SP, multivariate regression analysis revealed that OP was significantly associated with SP occurrence within 4 years (odds ratio, 2.99; 95% confidence interval, 1.46–6.12; $P < 0.01$), but the reciprocal relationship was not significantly observed (2.11; 0.59–7.59; $P = 0.25$) [13].

5.3 Prevalence of Symptom of Locomotive Organ Diseases, Such as Knee Pain and Lumbar Pain

The prevalence of knee pain and lumbar pain was determined from the survey results of the longitudinal cohorts of motor system organ (LOCOMO) study [15]. The LOCOMO study was initiated in 2008 through a grant from the Ministry of Health, Labour, and Welfare in Japan to integrate information from several cohorts established for the prevention of locomotive organ diseases. The LOCOMO study integrated information of 12,019 participants (3959 men and 8060 women) in cohorts comprising nine communities located in Tokyo (two regions), Wakayama (two regions), Hiroshima, Niigata, Mie, Akita, and Gunma prefectures. The three communities from the ROAD study were also involved in the LOCOMO study. LOCOMO study participants were questioned about pain in both knees through the following questions: 'Have you experienced right knee pain on most days (and continuously on at least 1 day) in the past month, in addition to the current pain?' and 'Have you experienced left knee pain on most days (and continuously on at least 1 day) in the past month, in addition to the current pain?' Subjects who answered 'yes' were considered to have knee pain. The presence of lumbar pain was determined by asking the following question: 'Have you experienced lumbar pain on most days (and continuously on at least 1 day) in the past month, in addition to the current pain?' Subjects who answered 'yes' were considered to have lumbar pain.

Figure 5.7 shows the prevalence of knee pain and lumbar pain. The prevalence of knee pain was 32.7% (men, 27.9%; women, 35.1%) and that of lumbar pain was 37.7% (men, 34.2%; women, 39.4%) [16]. On the basis of the total age-sex distributions derived from the Japanese census in 2010 [16], our results estimate that 18,000,000 (7,100,000 men and 10,900,000 women) and 27,700,000 (12,100,000 men and 15,600,000 women) people aged ≥40 years would be affected by knee pain and lumbar pain, respectively.

Among the 9046 individuals who were surveyed for both regarding knee pain and lumbar pain at the baseline examination in each cohort, we noted that the prevalence of both knee pain and lumbar pain was 12.2% (men, 10.9%; women, 12.8%) [15]. The prevalence of the coexistence of knee and lumbar pain in participants aged <40, 40–49, 50–59, 60–69, 70–79, and ≥80 years was 4.0%, 4.8%, 7.4%, 13.0%, 13.3%, and 11.7%, respectively (6.1%, 5.3%, 6.0%, 10.0%, 11.5%, and

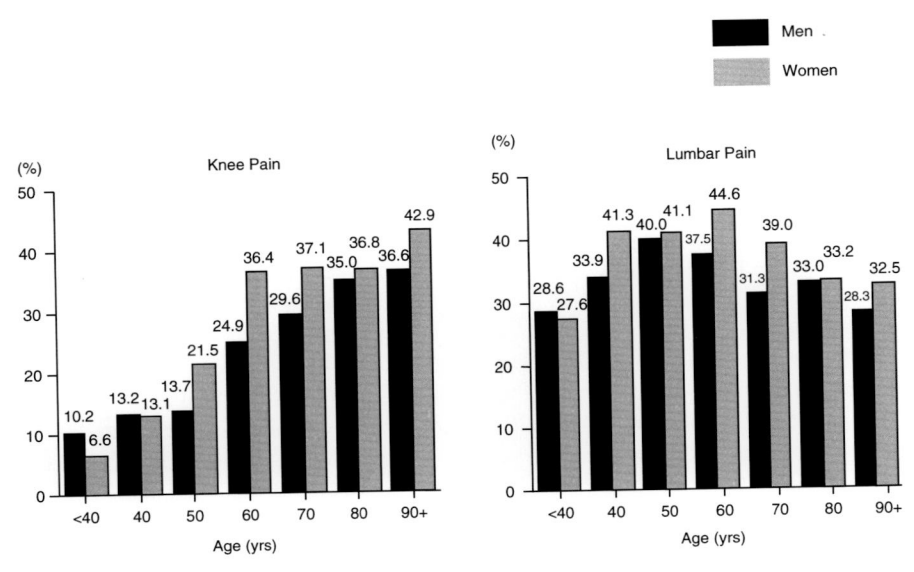

Fig. 5.7 Prevalence (%) of knee pain and lumbar pain. Yoshimura N, et al. J Bone Miner Metab 32: 524–532, 2014

13.2%, respectively, in men and 2.6%, 4.6%, 8.1%, 14.8%, 14.2%, and 11.0%, respectively, in women). On the basis of the total age-sex distributions derived from the Japanese census in 2010 [17], 6,800,000 people (2,800,000 men and 4,000,000 women) aged ≥40 years would be affected by both knee pain and lumbar pain.

5.4 Prevalence and Number of Patients with Locomotive Syndrome at Stages 1 and 2

As already mentioned, the JOA proposed three tests as candidate indices for assessing the risk of developing the locomotive syndrome and determined clinical decision limits for each of these [4]. The clinical decision limits were established in two stages as follows:

Stage 1 included (1) a two-step test score <1.3, (2) difficulty with one-leg standing from a 40-cm-high seat in the stand-up test (either leg), and (3) a 25-question GLFS score ≥7.

When a subject met any of the aforementioned conditions, s/he was diagnosed as starting to decline in mobility.

Stage 2 included (1) a two-step test score <1.1, (2) difficulty with standing from a 20-cm-high seat using both legs in the stand-up test, and (3) a 25-question GLFS score ≥16.

Any participant who met these conditions was diagnosed as progressing towards decline in mobility.

We used data from 1575 subjects (513 men and 1062 women) of the third survey who completed the stand-up test, two-step test, and 25-question GLFS for disability in mountainous and coastal areas.

Figure 5.8 shows the age-sex prevalence of the locomotive syndrome at stage 1. The prevalence was estimated at 69.8% (men, 68.4%; women, 70.5%) in the whole population. The prevalence tended to be significantly higher with age ($P < 0.001$), but there was no significant difference between the sexes ($P = 0.41$) [10].

Figure 5.9 shows the age-sex prevalence of the locomotive syndrome at stage 2 for which the prevalence was estimated at 25.1% (men, 22.7%; women, 26.3%). Again, the prevalence tended to be significantly higher with age ($P < 0.001$), but there was no significant difference between the sexes ($P = 0.13$) [10].

Combining these results with 2010 Japan census data [16], we estimated the number of potential locomotive syndrome patients. Thus, 45,900,000 (20,200,000 men and 25,700,000 women) and 13,800,000 people (4,600,000 men and 9,200,000 women) aged ≥40 years were categorised as potentially having locomotive syndrome stage 1 and stage 2, respectively.

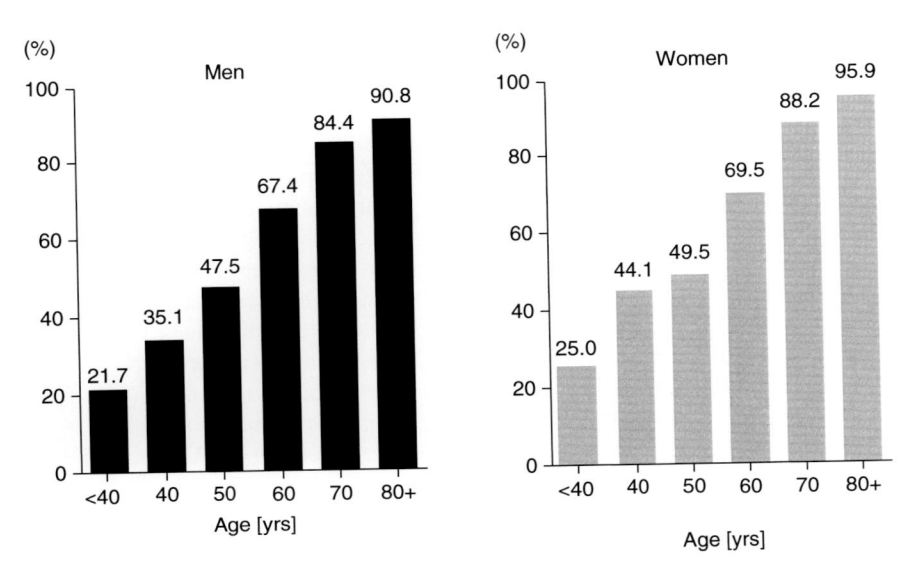

Fig. 5.8 Prevalence of locomotive syndrome in stage 1 based on clinical decision limits of three indices: the two-step test, stand-up test, and 25-question geriatric locomotive function scale. Yoshimura N, et al. Mod Rheumatol 27: 1–7, 2017

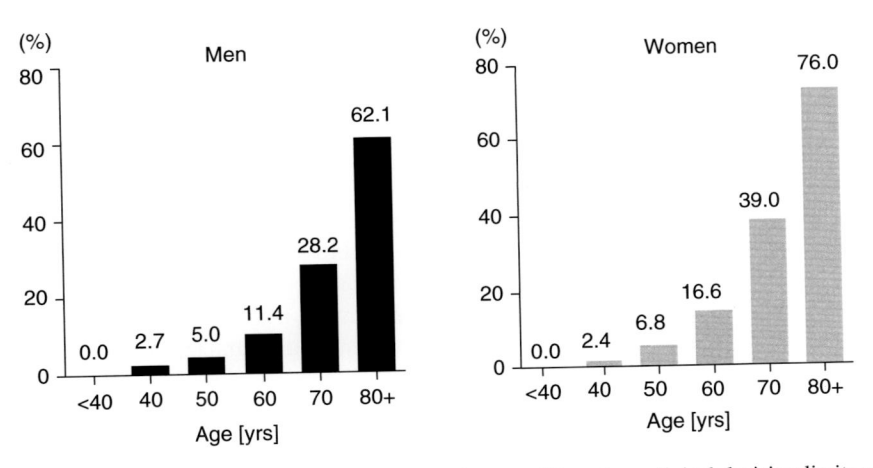

Fig. 5.9 Prevalence of the locomotive syndrome in stage 2 based on clinical decision limits of three indices: the two-step test, stand-up test, and 25-question geriatric locomotive function scale. Yoshimura N, et al. Mod Rheumatol 27: 1–7, 2017

5.5 Conclusion

Previously, there was little information regarding the epidemiology of locomotive organ disorders such as OA and OP and their symptoms such as knee and lumbar pain in Japan. The ROAD study is the first large observational study conducted in the Japanese population that was designed to supply essential information regarding OA and OP.

In this chapter, which uses the latest reports of population-based epidemiological studies such as the ROAD and LOCOMO studies, the prevalence of locomotive organ diseases, their symptoms, and locomotive syndrome at stages 1 and 2 were clarified. Determining the frequency of a disorder is the first step to preventing it. Hence, prevalence may be useful for determining a reduced target value in future interventional or observational studies with the aim of preventing disability among inhabitants in general. In addition, the prevalence of the coexistence of these diseases was very high. Therefore, there is an urgent need to draft and apply strategies for addressing the locomotive organ diseases that cause disability in the elderly.

Further, we clarified the age-sex distribution of the prevalence of locomotive syndrome stages 1 and 2 using the proposed clinical decision limits of three indices, including the two-step test, stand-up test, and 25-question GLFS. The estimated number of locomotive syndrome stage 1 patients (47,000,000 people) was very similar to that of individuals affected by either OA or OP [5]. In addition, one-fourth of subjects aged ≥40 were estimated to be progressing to decline in mobility. This proportion exponentially increased when only patients aged ≥70 years were considered. Since the population of Japan is ageing very rapidly, this distribution of stage 2 prevalence suggested that there is an urgent need to develop preventive strategies for addressing these diseases.

In conclusion, using the ROAD study data, we clarified the prevalence of KOA, LS, hip OA, OP, SP, knee and lumbar pain, and locomotive syndrome stages 1 and 2 and estimated the number of affected people in Japan. The study will provide the information required to develop clinical algorithms for the early identification of potential high-risk populations and policies for the detection and prevention of the locomotive syndrome. The knowledge gained from the large-scale population-based cohorts will have major implications for the understanding and management of several other issues associated with ageing.

Acknowledgments Excluding the authors, the results of the following ROAD study investigators are included in this manuscript: Drs. Shigeyuki Muraki and Toshiko Iidaka, Department of Preventive Medicine for Locomotive Organ Disorders, 22nd Century Medical and Research Center, The University of Tokyo; Hiroyuki Oka, Department of Medical Research and Management for Musculoskeletal Pain, 22nd Century Medical and Research Center, The University of Tokyo; Dr. Toru Akune, National Rehabilitation Center for Persons with Disabilities; and Dr. Hiroshi Kawaguchi, JCHO Tokyo Shinjuku Medical Center.

Conflict of Interest None to declare.

References

1. Ministry of Health, Labour, and Welfare. The outline of the results of National Livelihood Survey. 2016. http://www.mhlw.go.jp/toukei/saikin/hw/k-tyosa/k-tyosa16/dl/06.pdf.
2. Nakamura K. A 'super-aged' society and the 'locomotive syndrome'. J Orthop Sci. 2008;13:1–2.
3. Locomotive syndrome. In: Locomotive Challenge Council, editor. Locomotive syndrome pamphlet 2013. Tokyo: Japanese Orthopaedic Association; 2013.
4. Locomotive syndrome (in Japanese). In: Locomotive Challenge Council, editor. Locomotive syndrome pamphlet 2015. Tokyo: Japanese Orthopaedic Association; 2015.
5. Yoshimura N, Muraki S, Oka H, Mabuchi A, En-yo Y, Yoshida M, et al. Prevalence of knee osteoarthritis, lumbar spondylosis and osteoporosis in Japanese men and women: the research on osteoarthritis/osteoporosis against disability study. J Bone Miner Metab. 2009;27:620–8.
6. Yoshimura N, Muraki S, Oka H, Kawaguchi H, Nakamura K, Akune T. Cohort profile: research on osteoarthritis/osteoporosis against disability (ROAD) study. Int J Epidemiol. 2010;39:988–95.
7. Kellgren JH, Lawrence LS. Radiological assessment of osteo-arthrosis. Ann Rheum Dis. 1957;16:494–502.
8. Iidaka T, Muraki S, Akune T, Oka H, Kodama R, Tanaka S, et al. Prevalence of radiographic hip osteoarthritis and its association with hip pain in Japanese men and women: the ROAD study. Osteoarthr Cartil. 2016;24:117–23.
9. Japanese Official Statistics, Ministry of Internal Affairs and Communications. Population Census. 2005. http://www.e-stat.go.jp/SG1/estat/GL08020101.do?_toGL08020101_&tstatCode=000001007251.
10. Yoshimura N, Muraki S, Nakamura K, Tanaka S. Epidemiology of the locomotive syndrome: the research on osteoarthritis/osteoporosis against disability study 2005-2015. Mod Rheumatol. 2017;27:1–7.
11. Orimo H, Hayashi Y, Fukunaga M, Sone T, Fujiwara S, Shiraki M, et al. Osteoporosis diagnostic criteria review committee: Japanese Society for Bone and Mineral Research. Diagnostic criteria for primary osteoporosis: year 2000 revision. J Bone Miner Metab. 2001;19:331–7.
12. Chen LK, Liu LK, Woo J, Assantachai P, Auyeung TW, Bahyah KS, Chou MY, Chen LY, Hsu PS, Krairit O, Lee JS, Lee WJ, Lee Y, Liang CK, Limpawattana P, Lin CS, Peng LN, Satake S, Suzuki T, Won CW, Wu CH, Wu SN, Zhang T, Zeng P, Akishita M, Arai H. Sarcopenia in Asia: consensus report of the Asian Working Group for Sarcopenia. J Am Med Dir Assoc. 2014;15:95–101.
13. Yoshimura N, Muraki S, Oka H, Iidaka T, Kodama R, Kawaguchi H, Nakamura K, Tanaka S, Akune T. Is osteoporosis a predictor for future sarcopenia, or vice-versa? Four-year observations between the second and third ROAD study surveys. Osteoporos Int. 2017;28:189–99.
14. Yoshimura N, Muraki S, Oka H, Tanaka S, Kawaguchi H, Nakamura K, Akune T. Mutual associations among musculoskeletal diseases and metabolic syndrome components: a 3-year follow-up of the ROAD study. Mod Rheumatol. 2015;25:38–48.
15. Yoshimura N, Akune T, Fujiwara S, Nishiwaki Y, Shimizu Y, Yoshida H, Sudo A, Omori G, Yoshida M, Shimokata H, Suzuki T, Muraki S, Oka H, Nakamura K. Prevalence of knee pain, lumbar pain and its co-existence in Japanese men and women: the longitudinal cohorts of motor system organ (LOCOMO) study. J Bone Miner Metab. 2014;32:524–32.
16. Portal site of Official Statistics of Japan. Population Census. 2010. http://www.e-stat.go.jp/SG1/estat/GL08020103.do?_toGL08020103_&tclassID=000001034991&cycleCode=0&requestSender=search.

Chapter 6
Epidemiology of Dementia in a Community: The Hisayama Study

Toshiharu Ninomiya

Abstract The prevalence of dementia has increased rapidly over the past two decades in Japan, with approximately 15% of people aged ≥65 years in 2012. This steep increase in prevalence may have been caused by the increasing incidence of dementia and the improvement of the survival rate of individuals with dementia, in addition to the rapid aging of the population. It is important to begin protecting the brain before developing any cognitive impairment, because the pathophysiological processes of dementia begin many years before the onset of symptoms. The prevention and optimal management of risk factors such as hypertension and diabetes, tobacco cessation, regular exercise, and favorable diets would be needed as early as possible in the life cycle for the effective prevention of late-life dementia in Japan.

Keywords Dementia · Alzheimer's disease · Vascular dementia · Epidemiology · Prospective study

Abbreviations

AD Alzheimer's disease
CI Confidence interval
HR Hazard ratio
VaD Vascular dementia

T. Ninomiya
Department of Epidemiology and Public Health, Graduate School of Medical Sciences, Kyushu University, Fukuoka, Japan
e-mail: nino@eph.med.kyushu-u.ac.jp

© Springer Nature Singapore Pte Ltd. 2019
M. Washio, C. Kiyohara (eds.), *Health Issues and Care System for the Elderly*,
Current Topics in Environmental Health and Preventive Medicine,
https://doi.org/10.1007/978-981-13-1762-0_6

6.1 Introduction

Dementia is a syndrome that affects memory, thinking, behavior, and the ability to perform everyday activities. The major subtypes of dementia in community-dwelling populations are Alzheimer's disease (AD) and vascular dementia (VaD). AD has traditionally been considered a primarily neurodegenerative disorder characterized by neuritic plaques and neurofibrillary tangles, which are, respectively, formed by an accumulation of amyloid beta-protein and abnormal phosphorylation of the tau protein in neurons. Vascular dementia (VaD) develops as a consequence of strokes or chronic brain ischemia generated by small vessel disease.

The number of people with dementia worldwide is currently estimated at 46.8 million; this number is expected to double to 74.7 million by 2030 and to more than triple to 131.5 million by 2050 [1]. The global costs of dementia are enormous and still inequitably distributed. In the United States (US) alone, the cost was estimated as $818 billion in 2015, with anticipated increases to US$ 1 trillion in 2018 and US$ 2 trillion by 2030 [1, 2]. These cost increases arise from the increase in the number of people with dementia and the per person costs, especially in high-income countries [2]. Therefore, dementia is widely acknowledged as a public health and social care priority worldwide. The identification of risk factors and preventative strategies for each subtype of dementia has become a topic of scientific and public interest.

The Hisayama study is an ongoing population-based prospective cohort study of cerebro-cardiovascular diseases in the town of Hisayama, which is adjacent to the Fukuoka metropolitan area in southern Japan [3]. According to the national census, the age and occupational distributions and the nutrient intake of residents in this town have been almost identical to those of Japan as a whole during the past 50 years. In addition, the screening surveys of dementia have been repeated every 6 or 7 years in the residents aged ≥65 years since 1985 in this study [4]. The objective of this article was to use the epidemiological findings from the Hisayama study to review the current burden of and risk factors for dementia in Japan.

6.2 The Burden of Dementia in Japan

Japan has the oldest population in the world; 26.7% of individuals were 65 or older in 2015, and the life expectancy at birth was 80.98 years for men and 87.14 years for women in 2016 [5]. A recent report from the Ministry of Health, Labour and Welfare of Japan estimated that approximately 4.6 million people in Japan had dementia in 2012, which is equivalent to 15% of people aged 65 years or older [6]. In the Hisayama study, five cross-sectional surveys of dementia were conducted among residents of a Japanese community, aged 65 years or older, in 1985, 1992, 1998, 2005, and 2012 to investigate trends in the prevalence of dementia and its subtypes [4]. The participant rates of these five surveys were more than 92% of town residents aged 65 years or older. The unadjusted prevalence of total dementia increased significantly with time

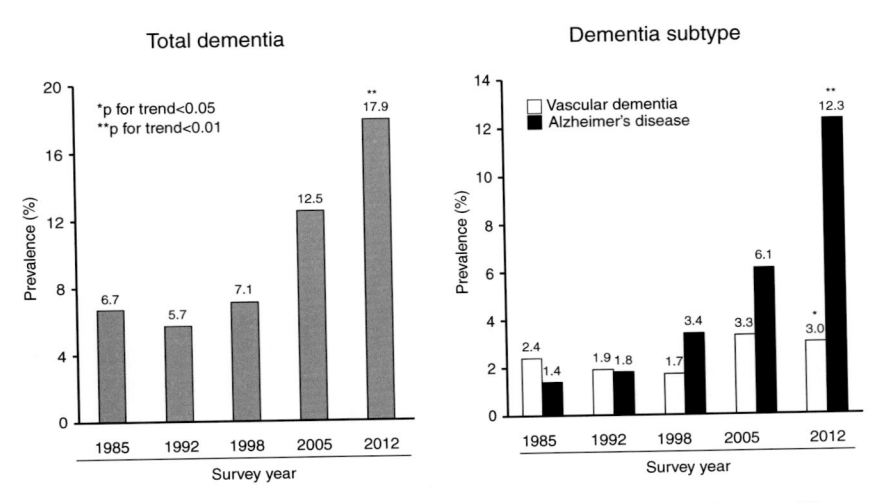

Fig. 6.1 Trend in prevalence of total dementia and its subtypes in the town of Hisayama. Hisayama residents, aged ≥65 years, unadjusted (cited by reference 4)

(6.7%, 5.7%, 7.1%, 12.5%, and 17.9%, respectively; P for trend <0.01) (Fig. 6.1). With regard to dementia subtypes, an increasing trend in the prevalence of AD was observed (1.4%, 1.8%, 3.4%, 6.1%, and 12.3%, respectively; P for trend <0.01), while the prevalence of VaD showed a decreasing trend between 1985 and 1998 and thereafter an increasing trend (2.4%, 1.9%, 1.7%, 3.3%, 3.0%, P for trend =0.02). Aging of the population is a major cause of the increase in the prevalence of dementia. However, after controlling for the confounding effects of aging, the upward trends in the prevalence of total dementia and AD remained significant, while the increasing trend in the prevalence of VaD disappeared. These findings suggest that the burden of dementia, especially AD, has increased rapidly over the past two decades in Japan.

To evaluate the change in the incidence of dementia with time, two different cohorts were established in the Hisayama study [4]. In 1988, a total of 837 residents aged ≥65 years participated in a screening survey (participation rate, 92%). After excluding subjects with dementia at baseline, the remaining total of 803 subjects were followed up for 10 years (the 1988 cohort). Similarly, 1231 subjects aged ≥65 years without dementia at baseline were followed up from 2002 to 2012 (the 2002 cohort). The incidence of total dementia and its subtypes were compared between the two cohorts.

The results showed that the incidence of total dementia increased significantly, by approximately 1.7-fold, between the 1988 and the 2002 cohort. With regard to dementia subtypes, the incidence of AD was 2.1-fold higher in the 2002 cohort than in the 1988 cohort (Fig. 6.2). There was no significant difference in the incidence of VaD between the two cohorts in either sex. The age-specific incidence of total dementia, AD, and VaD increased consistently with age in both cohorts. The age-specific incidence of total dementia and AD was marginally/significantly higher across the 65–84 year age groups in the 2002 cohort than that in the 1988 cohort, but

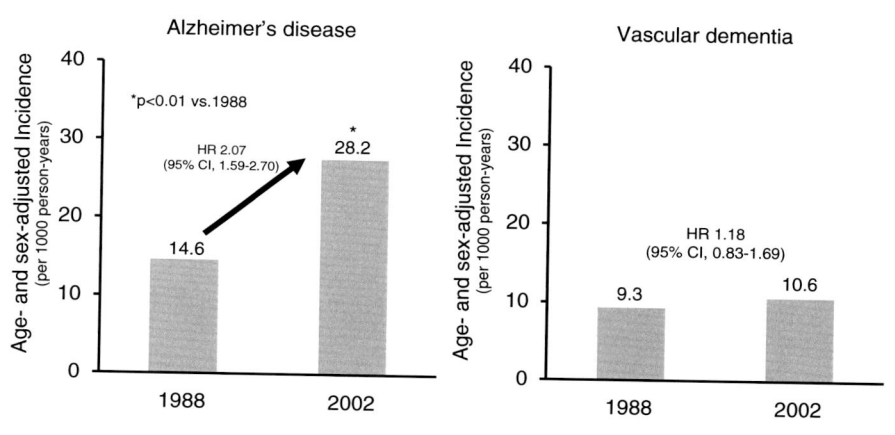

Fig. 6.2 Trend in age- and sex-adjusted incidence of dementia subtypes in the town of Hisayama. Hisayama residents, aged ≥65 years, 10-year follow-up. *HR* hazard ratio, *CI* confidence interval (cited by reference 4)

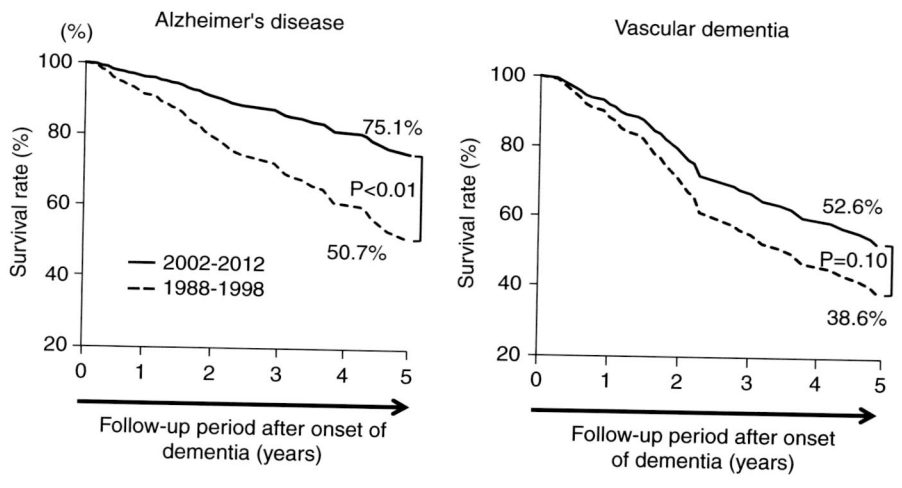

Fig. 6.3 Changes of age- and sex-adjusted survival rate of dementia subtypes after onset of dementia in the town of Hisayama. Hisayama residents, aged ≥65 years, 5-year follow-up (cited by reference 4)

no such trends were observed in the ≥85 years age group. However, the incidence of VaD did not change between the cohorts in any age group.

The increasing trend in the incidence of AD in Japan may be related to the recent increase in the burden of metabolic disorders such as diabetes or the spread of westernized lifestyle behaviors such as lack of exercise, which have been associated with higher risk of AD [7, 8]. In addition, the changes of the age- and sex-adjusted survival rates of each dementia subtype over 5 years after the onset of dementia were evaluated in the Hisayama study (Fig. 6.3) [4]. The estimated 5-year survival rate of all-cause dementia and AD improved from the 1988 cohort to the 2002 cohort (47.3% to 65.2% for all-cause dementia; 50.7% to 75.1% for AD; all $P < 0.01$), although the average age of onset of dementia was almost the same between the two cohorts (83 years in the 1988 cohort; 82 years in the 2002 cohort). A similar improvement of the 5-year survival rate of VaD was observed between the two cohorts (38.6% to 52.6%; $P = 0.10$). Together with progress in medical technology, the establishment of a public long-term care insurance system might help to improve the survival rate of dementia in Japan. These findings suggest that the recent increase in the prevalence of dementia in Japan derives from both an increased incidence of dementia and an improvement in the survival rates of dementia patients, in addition to the aging of the population in general. Therefore, there is a pressing need to build preventive strategies for dementia in Japan, as well to promote acceptance of dementia at the community level by disseminating relevant knowledge, improving attitudes, and enhancing social systems.

6.3 Risk Factors of Dementia

6.3.1 Hypertension

Hypertension has been recognized as one of the important risk factors for dementia. Because hypertension has also been shown to be a major risk factor for cerebrovascular disease, higher BP is likely to be strongly associated with a greater risk of VaD [9]. Moreover, some epidemiological studies have suggested that midlife hypertension is a risk factor for late-life dementia, whereas lower diastolic BP in late life may be related to increased risks of dementia and AD, which has traditionally been considered a primarily neurodegenerative disorder, although the results of observational longitudinal studies showing the effects of BP on the risks of dementia and its subtypes are inconsistent [10, 11]. These facts raise the possibilities that the effects of hypertension on the incidence of dementia may be different between midlife and late life, possibly because the longitudinal changes related to hypertension in the brain may begin earlier in the adult lifespan. Therefore, we investigated the association of BP levels in midlife and late life with the development of dementia and its subtypes in a general Japanese population.

A total of 668 community-dwelling Japanese individuals without dementia, aged 65 to 79 years, were followed up for 17 years, and the associations of late-life and midlife hypertension with the risk of VaD and AD were examined [12]. The age- and sex-adjusted incidence of VaD increased significantly with elevated late-life blood pressure levels (normal 2.3, prehypertension 8.4, stage 1 hypertension 12.6, and stage 2 hypertension 18.9 per 1000 person-years; P for trend <0.001). The subjects with prehypertension, stage 1, and stage 2 hypertension had 3.0-fold, 4.5-fold, and 5.6-fold greater risk of VaD, respectively, compared with normal-blood pressure subjects after adjusting for potential confounding factors (Fig. 6.4). Likewise, there was a positive association of midlife blood pressure levels with the risk of

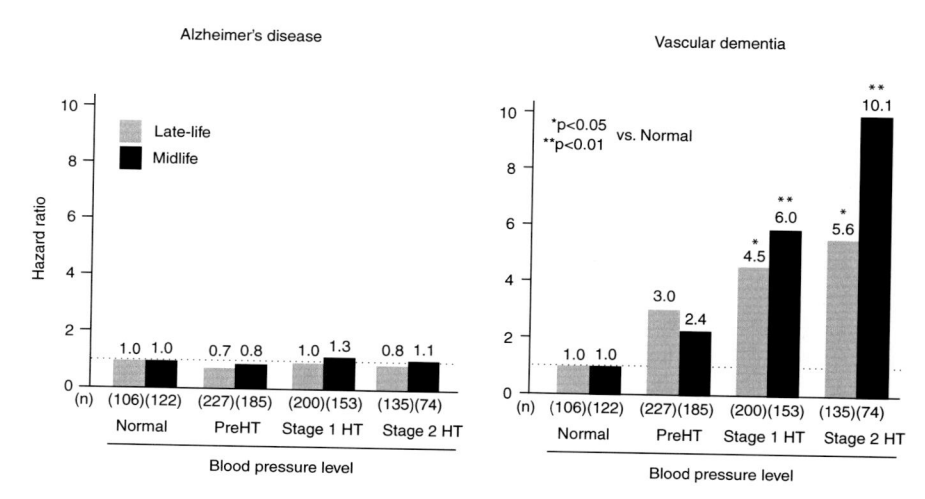

Fig. 6.4 Risks of dementia subtypes in people with late-life or midlife hypertension. 668 Hisayama residents aged 65–79 years, 1988–2005 and 534 residents aged 50–64 years, 1973–2005 (cited by reference 12). The hazard ratios were adjusted for age, sex, education level, antihypertensive agent use, diabetes, chronic kidney disease, serum total cholesterol, body mass index, history of stroke, smoking habits, and alcohol intake. *PreHT* prehypertension, *HT* hypertension

VaD. In contrast, there was no evidence of a significant association of midlife or late-life hypertension with the risk of AD (*P* for trend >0.4). In the analysis of the influence of changes in hypertension status from midlife to late life, the subjects with hypertension in midlife had an approximately fivefold greater risk of VaD than those without hypertension in both midlife and late life, irrespective of late-life blood pressure levels. Since higher BP causes small vessel disease and white matter lesions, long exposure to poorly controlled midlife hypertension presumably worsens arteriolosclerotic changes and lipohyalinosis in the deep subcortical white matter circuits [13–15]. This finding suggests that the vascular damages related to hypertension in the brain begin relatively early in the lifespan and gradually become less reversible. Therefore, it would be reasonable to suppose that the optimal control of midlife BP levels is clinically important in order to reduce the risk of late-life dementia in the general Japanese population.

6.3.2 Diabetes Mellitus

A number of population-based prospective studies have reported an association between diabetes mellitus and the development of dementia [16, 17]. In a meta-analysis, diabetes mellitus was associated with a 1.7-fold (95% confidence interval [CI] 1.5–1.8) greater risk of all dementia, without any heterogeneity in the magnitude of the association (I2 = 0.0%, *P* = 0.51) [16]. Substantially similar findings were observed in the subtypes of dementia, such as AD and VaD. The pooled hazard ratio (HR) for Alzheimer's disease in individuals with diabetes mellitus was 1.6 (95% CI 1.4–1.8). Similarly, a significant increase in the risk of vascular dementia was found with a pooled HR of 2.2 (95% CI 1.7–2.8). There were no evidences of heterogeneity in the association for either subtype of dementia across the studies (both I2 = 0.0%, $P > 0.4$). These findings provide evidence that subjects with diabetes mellitus have a 1.5- to 2.5-fold greater risk of dementia than those without it among community-dwelling elderly people.

In the Hisayama study, diabetes status was determined by oral glucose tolerance test, and dementia subtypes were diagnosed by detailed neurologic and morphologic examinations, including neuroimaging and autopsy. Intriguingly, this study revealed that greater 2-h postload plasma glucose (2-h PG) levels, but not greater fasting plasma glucose (FPG) levels, were linked to an increased risk of both AD and VaD in an elderly Japanese population [7]. The risk of AD almost doubled in those with 2-h PG of 7.8–11.0 mmol/L and tripled in those with 2-h PG above 11.0 mmol/L as compared with those with 2-h PG below 6.7 mmol/L (Fig. 6.5). These findings may suggest that hyperglycemia after glucose load is involved in the development of AD, as well as VaD.

The morphological changes of Alzheimer's disease occur in the hippocampus, amygdala, and medial temporal lobe in the early stages of the disease [18]. Patients in the early stage of AD have smaller volumes of the hippocampus and amygdala on MRI compared to healthy control subjects [19–21]. The results from the Rotterdam Scan Study showed that subjects with diabetes mellitus also had significantly lower volumes of the hippocampus and amygdala on MRI than subjects without diabetes mellitus [22]. In the Hisayama study, the association between diabetes and hippocampal atrophy was similarly investigated in 1238 community-dwelling Japanese

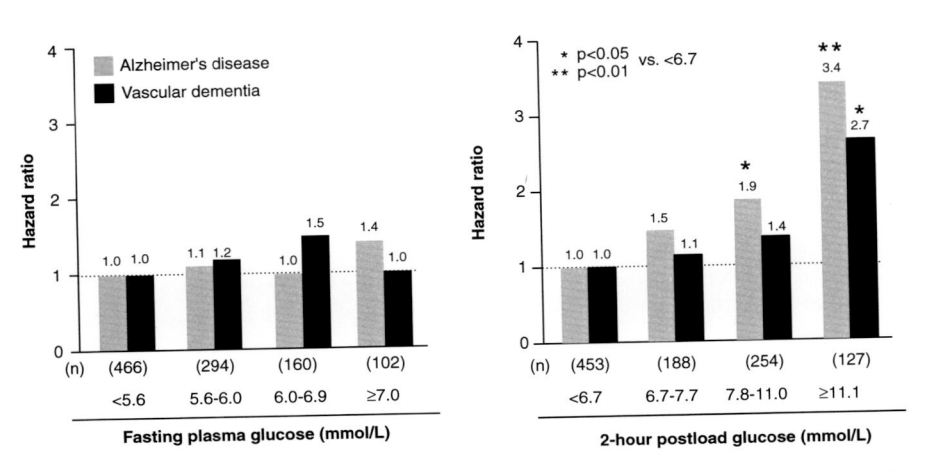

Fig. 6.5 Risk of dementia subtypes to the fasting and 2-h postload plasma glucose levels. 1017 Hisayama residents aged ≥60 years, 1988–2003 (cited by reference 7). The hazard ratios were adjusted for age, sex, education level, hypertension, serum total cholesterol, body mass index, waist-to-hip ratio, electrocardiogram abnormalities, history of stroke, smoking habits, alcohol intakes, and regular exercise

subjects aged 65 years or older who underwent brain MRI scans [23]. The results showed that diabetic subjects, especially those with higher 2-h PG levels, had a significantly lower hippocampal volume than nondiabetic subjects. Moreover, longer duration of diabetes was significantly associated with lower hippocampal volume. Thus subjects with diabetes in midlife had a greater risk of hippocampal atrophy than those with diabetes in late life.

Pathological analysis of the Hisayama data also showed a significant association between the diabetes-related factors and the neuropathology of Alzheimer's disease [24]. In this analysis, the risk of developing neuritic plaques increased significantly with elevations of 2-h PG levels, fasting insulin and the homeostasis model assessment of insulin resistance, but not with elevation of FPG levels after adjusting for confounding factors. The magnitudes of these associations were significantly greater in subjects with the APOEe4 allele than in those without. This suggests that hyperinsulinemia and insulin resistance may be involved in the etiology of Alzheimer's disease. The Honolulu Heart Program revealed that subjects with diabetes mellitus and the APOEe4 allele had a significantly higher odds ratio of the presence of hippocampal neuritic plaques and neurofibrillary tangles in the cortex and hippocampus than those with neither of these risk factors [25]. There were no clear associations between diabetes mellitus and these neuropathologies of AD in APOEe4 noncarriers.

These findings provide confirmatory evidence that diabetes mellitus is a significant risk factor for not only VaD but also AD. The etiology of cognitive impairments in subjects with diabetes mellitus is probably multifactorial, although the mechanisms underlying this association are not yet fully clarified. Since midlife diabetes has been associated with hippocampal atrophy, the optimal management of risk factors as early as possible in the life cycle may be important to prevent late-life dementia in subjects with diabetes mellitus.

6.3.3   Smoking

Smoking has been acknowledged to be a risk factor for dementia. A meta-analysis including 37 observational studies demonstrated that current smokers had a 30–40% increased risk of total dementia, AD, and VaD compared to never smokers [26]. On the other hand, the risk of dementia and its subtypes did not increase in ever smokers as compared with never smokers. In the Hisayama study, the association between midlife and late-life smoking and risk of dementia was investigated [27]. A total 754 subjects without dementia aged 65–84 in 1988 were followed up for 17 years, 619 of whom had participated in a health examination conducted in 1973–1974. Subjects with a smoking habit in both midlife and late life had a significantly greater multivariable-adjusted risk of total dementia (HR 2.3; 95% CI 1.5–3.5), AD (HR 2.0; 95% CI 1.1–3.6), and VaD (HR 2.9; 95% CI 1.3–6.2) compared to lifelong nonsmokers. Intriguingly, the risk of AD and VaD decreased in midlife smokers who quit smoking in late life. These findings suggest that persistent smoking from midlife to late life is a significant risk factor for dementia and its subtypes in the general Japanese population. Smoking cessation needs to become a priority for prevention of dementia, which is likely to play an important role in reducing risk of dementia.

6.3.4 Physical Activity

High physical activity has recently attracted attention as a protective factor against dementia. Several epidemiological studies have assessed the relationship between physical activity and risk of dementia [28]. A recent meta-analysis including 117,410 subjects from 45 longitudinal studies clearly demonstrated that high physical activity had a favorable effect on cognitive decline, yielding an approximately 30% risk reduction [28]. Moreover, subjects with high physical activity had a significantly 21% (95% CI 12–31%) lower risk of total dementia and a significantly 38% (95% CI 25–51%) lower risk of AD, but no significant relationship between physical activity and risk of VaD was observed. The findings from the Hisayama study also appeared to suggest a significant inverse association between physical activity and risk for total dementia, especially AD, in a 17-year prospective study of an elderly Japanese population [8]. Several animal and clinical studies have shown that high physical activity inhibits hippocampal atrophy and deposition of ß-amyloid in the brain, thereby conferring protection against dementia, especially AD [29–31]. In addition, several prospective studies have shown that physical activity may have a protective influence on the development of dementia via mental stimulation and psychosocial activities [32]. These findings suggest that physical activity would be strongly recommended in order to prevent the future development of AD.

6.3.5 Diet

A number of previous epidemiological studies addressed effects of the Mediterranean dietary pattern on risk of dementia and showed that higher intakes of vegetables, fruits, and fish were linked to lower risk of dementia [33]. Gu et al. assessed the dietary pattern associated with the incidence of dementia in a US population, with the result that the extracted dietary pattern was positively correlated with high intake of salad dressing, nuts, tomatoes, poultry, cruciferous vegetables, fruits, and dark green leafy vegetables and negatively correlated with high-fat dairy, red meat, organ meat, and butter, and a greater adherence to this dietary pattern was associated with a lower risk of dementia [34].

Only a few epidemiological studies have attempted to investigate the association between diet and the development of dementia in Japanese populations. The findings from the Hisayama study showed that higher self-reported dietary intakes of potassium, calcium, and magnesium reduced the risk of total dementia and VaD, but not of AD, in 1081 community-dwelling Japanese individuals without dementia aged 60 years and older during a 17-year follow-up [35]. The intakes of minerals were calculated by using a 70-item semiquantitative food frequency questionnaire and were divided into quartiles. The multivariable-adjusted HRs for total dementia were 0.5 (95% CI 0.3–0.9), 0.6 (95% CI 0.4–1.0), and 0.6 (95% CI 0.4–1.0) for the highest quartiles of potassium, calcium, and magnesium intake, respectively, as compared with the lowest quartiles. There is also some epidemiological evidence that these minerals have favorable effects against cerebrovascular disease, possibly through an improvement of hypertension, dyslipidemia, and insulin resistance [36, 37]. In the present analysis, subjects in the highest quartiles of these minerals tended to eat more potatoes, soybeans and soybean products, vegetables, fruits and fruit juices, algae, fish, eggs, and milk and dairy products and had less rice, meat, sugar, and alcoholic beverages. Moreover, this study also identified a dietary pattern associated with lower risk of dementia in 1006 community-dwelling Japanese individuals without dementia aged 60–79 years during a 17-year follow-up [38]. The dietary pattern was characterized by a high intake of soybeans and soybean products, green vegetables, other vegetables, algae, milk and dairy products, potatoes, fruits and fruit juices, and fish and a low intake of rice and alcohol. The multivariable-adjusted risk of total dementia decreased by 30% (HR 0.7, 95% CI 0.5–0.9) in subjects with the highest quartile of scores for this dietary pattern as compared with those with the lowest quartile. With regard to subtypes of dementia, individuals with the highest quartile of scores for this dietary pattern had a significantly lower risk of either AD (HR 0.7; 95% CI 0.4–1.1) or VaD (HR 0.5; 95% CI 0.2–0.9). Despite the different dietary customs among various populations, the dietary patterns and food groups detected are substantially similar.

6.4 Conclusions

Our findings indicated that the prevalence of dementia, especially AD, increased greatly over the past quarter century in a general population of Japanese elderly. This steep increase in prevalence may have been caused by the increasing incidence of dementia and the improvement of the survival rate of individuals with dementia, in addition to the rapid aging of the population. It is greatly to be hoped that new and effective drugs will be developed for the treatment of dementia, but no definitive evidence of any effective pharmacological treatment for dementia exists so far. Since the pathophysiological processes of dementia begin many years before any symptoms appear, it is crucial to begin protecting the brain before any cognitive impairment becomes manifest. The prevention and optimal management of risk factors such as hypertension and diabetes, tobacco cessation, regular exercise, and favorable diets would be needed as early as possible in the life cycle for the effective prevention of late-life dementia in Japan. Further research should attempt to explore effective preventive and/or therapeutic strategies against dementia.

Conflict of Interest/Disclosure None.

References

1. The World Alzheimer Report, 2015. The global impact of dementia. https://www.alz.co.uk/research/WorldAlzheimerReport2015.pdf.
2. Wimo A, Guerchet M, Ali GC, Wu YT, Prina AM, Winblad B, Jönsson L, Liu Z, Prince M. The worldwide costs of dementia 2015 and comparisons with 2010. Alzheimers Dement. 2017;13:1–7.
3. Hata J, Ninomiya T, Hirakawa Y, Nagata M, Mukai N, Gotoh S, Fukuhara M, Ikeda F, Shikata K, Yoshida D, Yonemoto K, Kamouchi M, Kitazono T, Kiyohara Y. Secular trends in cardiovascular disease and its risk factors in Japanese: half-century data from the Hisayama Study (1961-2009). Circulation. 2013;128:1198–205.
4. Ohara T, Hata J, Yoshida D, Mukai N, Nagata M, Iwaki T, Kitazono T, Kanba S, Kiyohara Y, Ninomiya T. Trends in dementia prevalence, incidence, and survival rate in a Japanese community. Neurology. 2017;88:1925–32.
5. Cabinet Office Government of Japan. Annual Report on the Aging Society, 2016. http://www8.cao.go.jp/kourei/english/annualreport/2016/pdf/c1-1.pdf.
6. Ministry of Health, Labour and Welfare of Japan. Abridged Life Tables for Japan. 2016. http://www.mhlw.go.jp/english/database/db-hw/lifetb16/dl/lifetb16-01.pdf.
7. Ohara T, Doi Y, Ninomiya T, Hirakawa Y, Hata J, Iwaki T, Kanba S, Kiyohara Y. Glucose tolerance status and risk of dementia in the community: the Hisayama study. Neurology. 2011;77:1126–34.
8. Kishimoto H, Ohara T, Hata J, Ninomiya T, Yoshida D, Mukai N, Nagata M, Ikeda F, Fukuhara M, Kumagai S, Kanba S, Kitazono T, Kiyohara Y. The long-term association between physical activity and risk of dementia in the community: the Hisayama Study. Eur J Epidemiol. 2016;31:267–74.
9. Fratiglioni L, Launer LJ, Andersen K, Breteler MM, Copeland JR, Dartigues JF, Lobo A, Martinez-Lage J, Soininen H, Hofman A. Incidence of dementia and major subtypes in Europe: a collaborative study of population-based cohorts. Neurologic Diseases in the Elderly Research Group. Neurology. 2000;54(11 Suppl 5):S10–5.
10. Qiu C, Winblad B, Fratiglioni L. The age-dependent relation of blood pressure to cognitive function and dementia. Lancet Neurol. 2005;4:487–99.
11. Elias PK, Elias MF, Robbins MA, Budge MM. Blood pressure-related cognitive decline: does age make a difference? Hypertension. 2004;44:631–6.
12. Ninomiya T, Ohara T, Hirakawa Y, Yoshida D, Doi Y, Hata J, Kanba S, Iwaki T, Kiyohara Y. Midlife and late-life blood pressure and dementia in Japanese elderly: the Hisayama study. Hypertension. 2011;58:22–8.
13. Swan GE, DeCarli C, Miller BL, Reed T, Wolf PA, Jack LM, Carmelli D. Association of midlife blood pressure to late-life cognitive decline and brain morphology. Neurology. 1998;51:986–93.
14. Dufouil C, de Kersaint-Gilly A, Besançon V, Levy C, Auffray E, Brunnereau L, Alpérovitch A, Tzourio C. Longitudinal study of blood pressure and white matter hyperintensities: the EVA MRI Cohort. Neurology. 2001;56:921–6.
15. Birns J, Markus H, Kalra L. Blood pressure reduction for vascular risk: is there a price to be paid? Stroke. 2005;36:1308–13.
16. Ninomiya T. Diabetes mellitus and dementia. Curr Diab Rep. 2014;14:487.
17. Chatterjee S, Peters SA, Woodward M, Mejia Arango S, Batty GD, Beckett N, Beiser A, Borenstein AR, Crane PK, Haan M, Hassing LB, Hayden KM, Kiyohara Y, Larson EB, Li CY, Ninomiya T, Ohara T, Peters R, Russ TC, Seshadri S, Strand BH, Walker R, Xu W, Huxley RR. Type 2 diabetes as a risk factor for dementia in women compared with men: a pooled analysis of 2.3 million people comprising more than 100,000 cases of dementia. Diabetes Care. 2016;39:300–7.
18. Braak H, Braak E. Neuropathological stageing of Alzheimer-related changes. Acta Neuropathol. 1991;82:239–59.

19. Convit A, De Leon MJ, Tarshish C, De Santi S, Tsui W, Rusinek H, George A. Specific hippocampal volume reductions in individuals at risk for Alzheimer's disease. Neurobiol Aging. 1997;18:131–8.
20. Schott JM, Fox NC, Frost C, Scahill RI, Janssen JC, Chan D, Jenkins R, Rossor MN. Assessing the onset of structural change in familial Alzheimer's disease. Ann Neurol. 2003;53: 181–8.
21. Krasuski JS, Alexander GE, Horwitz B, Daly EM, Murphy DG, Rapoport SI, Schapiro MB. Volumes of medial temporal lobe structures in patients with Alzheimer's disease and mild cognitive impairment (and in healthy controls). Biol Psychiatry. 1998;43: 60–8.
22. den Heijer T, Vermeer SE, van Dijk EJ, Prins ND, Koudstaal PJ, Hofman A, Breteler MM. Type 2 diabetes and atrophy of medial temporal lobe structures on brain MRI. Diabetologia. 2003;46:1604–10.
23. Hirabayashi N, Hata J, Ohara T, Mukai N, Nagata M, Shibata M, Gotoh S, Furuta Y, Yamashita F, Yoshihara K, Kitazono T, Sudo N, Kiyohara Y, Ninomiya T. Association between diabetes and hippocampal atrophy in elderly Japanese: the Hisayama study. Diabetes Care. 2016;39:1543–14549.
24. Matsuzaki T, Sasaki K, Tanizaki Y, Hata J, Fujimi K, Matsui Y, Sekita A, Suzuki SO, Kanba S, Kiyohara Y, Iwaki T. Insulin resistance is associated with the pathology of Alzheimer disease: the Hisayama study. Neurology. 2010;75:764–70.
25. Peila R, Rodriguez BL, Launer LJ. Type 2 diabetes, apoe gene, and the risk for dementia and related pathologies: the Honolulu-Asia aging study. Diabetes. 2002;51:1256–62.
26. Zhong G, Wang Y, Zhang Y, Guo JJ, Zhao Y. Smoking is associated with an increased risk of dementia: a meta-analysis of prospective cohort studies with investigation of potential effect modifiers. PLoS One. 2015;10:e0118333.
27. Ohara T, Ninomiya T, Hata J, Ozawa M, Yoshida D, Mukai N, Nagata M, Iwaki T, Kitazono T, Kanba S, Kiyohara Y. Midlife and late-life smoking and risk of dementia in the community: the Hisayama study. J Am Geriatr Soc. 2015;63:2332–9.
28. Guure CB, Ibrahim NA, Adam MB, Said SM. Impact of physical activity on cognitive decline, dementia, and its subtypes: meta-analysis of prospective studies. Biomed Res Int. 2017;2017:9016924.
29. Erickson KI, Voss MW, Prakash RS, Basak C, Szabo A, Chaddock L, et al. Exercise training increases size of hippocampus and improves memory. Proc Natl Acad Sci U S A. 2011;108:3017–22.
30. Adlard PA, Perreau VM, Pop V, Cotman CW. Voluntary exercise decreases amyloid load in a transgenic model of Alzheimer's disease. J Neurosci. 2005;25:4217–21.
31. Liu HL, Zhao G, Zhang H, Shi LD. Long-term treadmill exercise inhibits the progression of Alzheimer's disease-like neuropathology in the hippocampus of APP/PS1 transgenic mice. Behav Brain Res. 2013;256:261–72.
32. Karp A, Paillard-Borg S, Wang HX, Silverstein M, Winblad B, Fratiglioni L. Mental, physical and social components in leisure activities equally contribute to decrease dementia risk. Dement Geriatr Cogn Disord. 2006;21:65–73.
33. Psaltopoulou T, Sergentanis TN, Panagiotakos DB, Sergentanis IN, Kosti R, Scarmeas N. Mediterranean diet, stroke, cognitive impairment, and depression: A meta-analysis. Ann Neurol. 2013;74:580–91.
34. Gu Y, Nieves JW, Stern Y, Luchsinger JA, Scarmeas N. Food combination and Alzheimer disease risk: a protective diet. Arch Neurol. 2010;67:699–706.
35. Ozawa M, Ninomiya T, Ohara T, Hirakawa Y, Doi Y, Hata J, Uchida K, Shirota T, Kitazono T, Kiyohara Y. Self-reported dietary intake of potassium, calcium, and magnesium and risk of dementia in the Japanese: the Hisayama study. J Am Geriatr Soc. 2012;60: 1515–20.

36. Larsson SC, Virtanen MJ, Mars M, Mannisto S, Pietinen P, Albanes D, Virtamo J. Magnesium, calcium, potassium, and sodium intakes and risk of stroke in male smokers. Arch Intern Med. 2008;168:459–65.
37. Iso H, Stampfer MJ, Manson JE, Rexrode K, Hennekens CH, Colditz GA, Speizer FE, Willett WC. Prospective study of calcium, potassium, and magnesium intake and risk of stroke in women. Stroke. 1999;30:1772–9.
38. Ozawa M, Ninomiya T, Ohara T, Doi Y, Uchida K, Shirota T, Yonemoto K, Kitazono T, Kiyohara Y. Dietary patterns and risk of dementia in an elderly Japanese population: the Hisayama study. Am J Clin Nutr. 2013;97:1076–82.

Chapter 7
Obesity and Diabetes Mellitus as Risk Factors for Cardiovascular Disease in the Elderly

Hirofumi Ohnishi and Shigeyuki Saitoh

Abstract In recent years, the prevalence of obesity has been increasing in older people with aging of the population. Obesity is the most important risk factor for several lifestyle-related diseases including type 2 diabetes, hypertension, and cardiovascular disease in the elderly population as well as in the middle-aged population. However, the impact of obesity on incidence of lifestyle-related diseases and all-cause or cardiovascular disease (CVD) mortality is weaker in the elderly population than in the younger population. It is also known that the relationship between waist circumference and CVD mortality in men aged ≤ 65 years is U-shaped. Consideration of the different effects of obesity on lifestyle-related diseases in elderly and non-elderly people may be important for the prevention of lifestyle-related diseases.

The epidemic of diabetes mellitus in the elderly is an important global problem as well as obesity. Elderly patients with type 2 diabetes are more likely than middle-aged patients to have diabetic microangiopathy and macroangiopathy, and poorly controlled diabetes is one of the strong risk factors for CVD or all-cause death in the elderly population as well as in the middle-aged population. However, several studies have shown that there is a J-curve phenomenon in the relationship between HbA1c and CVD events or all-cause mortality in elderly patients with type 2 diabetes. Intensive control of diabetes mellitus causes severe hypoglycemia, and severe hypoglycemia may increase CVD events in the elderly individuals with diabetes mellitus. We have to achieve both maintenance of a good control level of blood glucose to avoid long-term complications and minimization of hypoglycemia and hypoglycemia-associated morbidity and mortality.

H. Ohnishi (✉)
Department of Public Health, Sapporo Medical University School of Medicine, Sapporo, Hokkaido, Japan
e-mail: hohnishi@sapmed.ac.jp

S. Saitoh
Department of Basics and Clinical Medicine, Sapporo Medical University School of Health Sciences, Sapporo, Hokkaido, Japan

© Springer Nature Singapore Pte Ltd. 2019
M. Washio, C. Kiyohara (eds.), *Health Issues and Care System for the Elderly*,
Current Topics in Environmental Health and Preventive Medicine,
https://doi.org/10.1007/978-981-13-1762-0_7

Keywords Obesity · Diabetes mellitus · Cardiovascular disease · All-cause death · Sarcopenic obesity · Hypoglycemia · J-curve phenomenon

7.1 Obesity in the Elderly and Lifestyle-Related Diseases or Cardiovascular Disease

In recent years, the prevalence of obesity in older people has increased with aging of the population in developed countries. In the United States, more than 30% of men and women aged 60 years or over are obese as defined by a body mass index (BMI) of 30 kg/m^2 or more [1]. In Japan, the National Health and Nutrition Survey in 2015 showed that the prevalences of obesity defined as a BMI of 25 kg/m^2 or more were 28% and 25% in men and women aged 60 years or over, respectively. Although the cutoff points of BMI are different in Asian and Western countries, an epidemic of obesity is an important and common global problem.

Obesity is the most important risk factor for several lifestyle-related diseases in the elderly population as well as in the middle-aged population. In fact, BMI and waist circumference have been shown to be strongly associated with the prevalences and incidences of type 2 diabetes, hypertension, and dyslipidemia [2–4]. Moreover, obesity is recognized as a risk factor for cardiovascular disease (CVD) and all-cause death. However, the impact of obesity on the incidences of lifestyle-related diseases and all-cause or CVD mortality is less in the older population than in the younger population.

We have reported the effect of abdominal obesity (AO) on new onset of type 2 diabetes in a general Japanese elderly population compared with that in a non-elderly population [5]. We have been carrying out a cohort study in two towns in Hokkaido, called "The Tanno-Sobetsu study", for more than 40 years and have reported risk factors for various lifestyle-related diseases and cardiovascular disease [3, 4, 6]. The participants in the study were 827 people aged 29–84 years who underwent medical examinations in 1994 and subsequently in either 2003 or 2004, after the exclusion of individuals with type 2 diabetes at baseline. The participants were divided into two groups according to waist circumference at baseline using the Japanese cutoff points: an AO group (waist circumferences of 85 cm or more for men and 90 cm or more for women) and a non-AO group. The percentages of individuals with new onset of type 2 diabetes recorded in either in 2003 or 2004 were compared between these two groups, and the odds ratio (OR) of AO for new onset of type 2 diabetes was calculated separately for elderly ($\geq$65 years of age) and non-elderly (<65 years of age) participants using multiple logistic regression analysis. The percentage of non-elderly participants with new onset of type 2 diabetes was significantly higher in the AO group than in the non-AO group (16.9% vs. 5.4%), but there was no statistically significant difference between the elderly participants in the two groups (12.7% vs. 7.1%). Multiple logistic regression analysis showed that there was a significant relationship between AO and NODM (OR, 2.68; 95% confidence interval (CI), 1.05–6.90) in the non-elderly subjects but not in the elderly subjects (OR, 0.67; 95% CI, 0.16–2.84). Consideration of the dif-

Table. 7.1 Comparisons of odds ratios of the existence of abdominal obesity for new onset of type 2 diabetes in non-elderly and elderly individuals [5]

	Model 1	Model 2	Model 3
Non-elderly (<65 years)	3.67 (95% CI, 1.67–8.27)	3.72 (95% CI, 1.59–8.67)	2.68 (95% CI, 1.05–6.90)
Elderly (≥65 years)	1.47 (95% CI, 0.47–4.59)	1.60 (95% CI, 0.49–5.19)	0.67 (95% CI, 0.16–2.84)

Model 1: Adjusted for age and gender
Model 2: Model 1 + total cholesterol, systolic blood pressure, smoking, and family history of diabetes mellitus
Model 3: Model 2 + fasting plasma glucose ≥110 mg/dL at baseline

ferent effects of AO on new onset of type 2 diabetes in elderly and non-elderly people may be important for the prevention of type 2 diabetes (Table 7.1).

To clarify the association between waist circumference and risk of all-cause or cardiovascular mortality in the Japanese population, we conducted pooled analysis of data from Japanese community-based studies including our cohort data [7]. A total of 3554 men and 4472 women who had no history of CVD were registered from 3 cohorts, and their waist circumferences were measured at baseline during the period from 1988 to 1996. Endpoints were all-cause death and CVD death, and the participants were followed up for 14.7 years. Hazard ratios (HRs) were calculated using the Cox proportional hazards model and a penalized spline method, after adjustment for the study cohort, age, smoking, alcohol drinking, hypertension, dyslipidemia, and diabetes. The highest quintile of waist circumference in men was associated with a linear reduction in all-cause mortality risk compared with the lowest quintile (HR, 0.73; 95% CI, 0.60–0.89; P for trend = 0.001). When stratifying participants according to age, CVD mortality risk was increased in men aged ≤65 years with a larger waist circumference. This relationship was U-shaped. On the other hand, in men aged >65 years, waist circumference was associated with all-cause mortality rather than CVD mortality (Fig. 7.1). In women, waist circumference was not associated with all-cause or CVD mortality risk.

A similar association was observed in a previous study. Hildrum et al. reported the relationship between metabolic syndrome and risk of mortality in middle-aged versus elderly individuals [8]. A total of 6748 men and women who participated in the Nord-Trøndelag Health Study, Norway, from 1995 to 1997 (HUNT 2) were followed up for 7.9 years. In individuals who were 40–59 years of age at baseline, the hazard ratios of metabolic syndrome defined by the International Diabetes Federation criteria for cardiovascular mortality and all-cause mortality were 3.97 (95% CI, 2.00–7.88) and 2.06 (95% CI, 1.35–3.13), respectively. After the age of 60 years, metabolic syndrome was not associated with increased mortality rates. These data suggest that the contribution of abdominal obesity to new onset of type 2 diabetes and CVD mortality may be small in the older population than in the younger population. Therefore, from the viewpoint of prevention of type 2 diabetes or CVD events, lifestyle intervention to lose body weight may be more effective for young- and middle-aged people than for elderly people. Moreover, from the

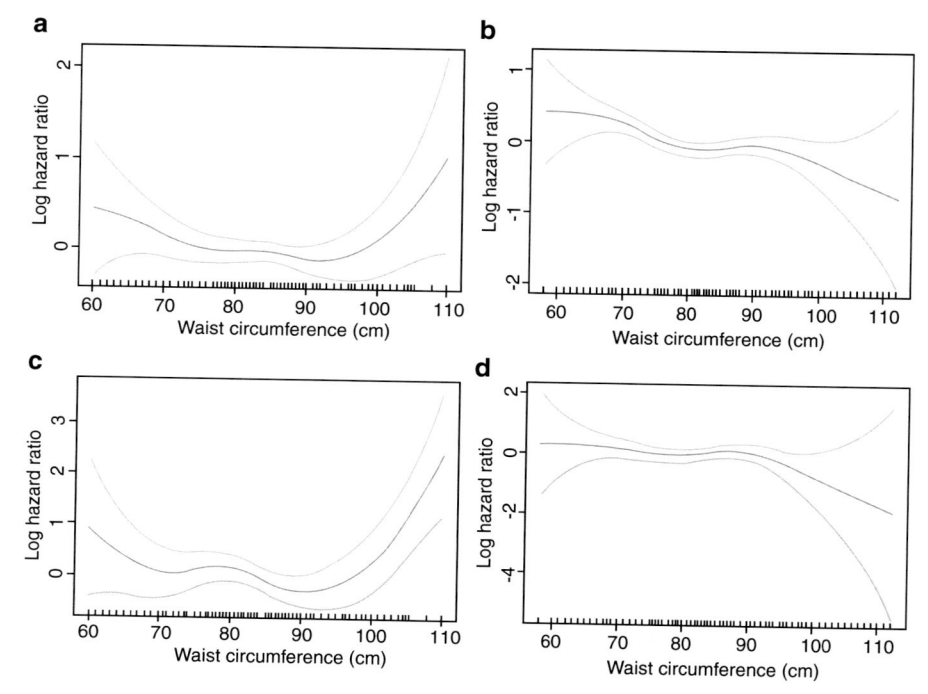

Fig. 7.1 P-spline fitting curves of hazard ratios and 95% confidence intervals for all-cause and cardiovascular disease deaths vs. waist circumference in men <65 years and ≥65 years of age. (**a**) All-cause death, age <65 years (nonlinear trend, $P = 0.089$); (**b**) all-cause death, age ≥65 years ($P = 0.11$); (**c**) CVD death, age <65 years ($P < 0.001$); (**d**) CVD death, age ≥65 years ($P = 0.31$). The hazard ratios were adjusted for age, study community, smoking habits, alcohol consumption, hypertension, hyperlipidemia, and diabetes mellitus. Actual waist circumference used in the present analysis is marked on the x-axis [7]

viewpoint of decrease in all-cause mortality in the elderly, we may have to intervene for individuals with low BMI using nutritional guidance by dieticians.

A state of having both sarcopenia and obesity is known as sarcopenic obesity [9]. Sarcopenic obesity cannot be assessed by only BMI because it consists of both an increase in body fat and decrease in muscle mass. Body composition that includes body fat and muscle mass is commonly measured using dual energy X-ray absorption (DXA) or bioelectrical impedance analysis (BIA), and obesity is commonly defined according to BMI, percentage of body fat, and waist circumference. Based on the existence of sarcopenia and obesity, the elderly population can be divided into four categories: non-sarcopenia and non-obesity (NS-NO), non-sarcopenia and obesity (NS-O), sarcopenia and non-obesity (S-NO), and sarcopenia and obesity (S-O, i.e., sarcopenic obesity). Several studies have shown differences in the prevalences and incidences of dyslipidemia, hypertension, and metabolic syndrome among these four categories in the elderly population. Baek et al. reported that sarcopenic obesity was associated with an increased risk for dyslipidemia in Korean elderly men according to the 2008–2010 Korea National Health and Nutrition Examination Survey

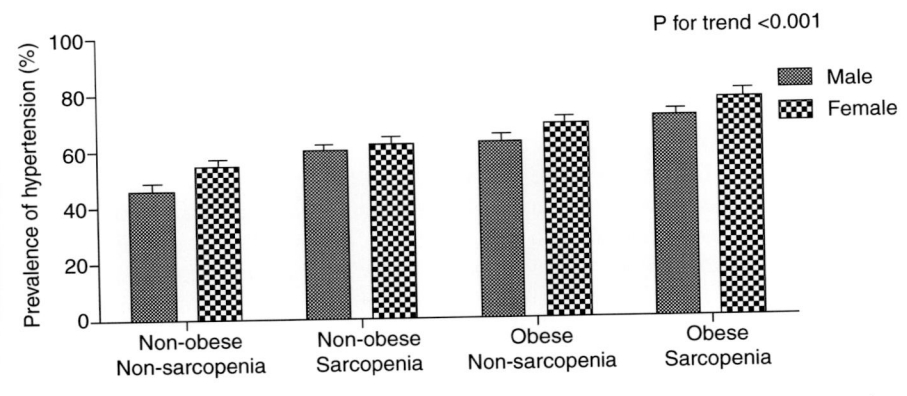

Fig. 7.2 Prevalence of hypertension according to the four body composition categories based on obesity and sarcopenia. In both the obese and non-obese groups, subjects with sarcopenia had a higher prevalence of hypertension than did subjects without sarcopenia [11]

(KNHANES) [10]. The odds ratio (OR) for dyslipidemia was higher in the S-O group (OR, 2.82; 95% CI, 1.76–4.51) than in the NS-O group (OR, 2.12; 95% CI, 1.11–4.07) and the S-NO group (OR, 1.46; 95% CI, 1.01–2.11). In another analysis based on data of the KNHANES 2008–2010 [11], sarcopenic obesity was more strongly associated with hypertension than was simply obesity or sarcopenia (Fig. 7.2). After adjustment for several confounding factors, the ORs for having hypertension were 1.5 (95% CI, 1.23–1.84) in the S-NO group, 2.08 (95% CI, 1.68–2.57) in the NS-O group, and 3.0 (95% CI, 2.48–3.63) in the S-O group, compared with the NS-NO group. Another study including a total of 600 community-dwelling individuals in Northern Taiwan showed the relationship between sarcopenic obesity and metabolic syndrome defined by the consensus of National Cholesterol Education Program Adult Treatment Panel III modified for Asians [12]. The ORs for having metabolic syndrome were 1.98 (95% CI, 1.25–3.16) in the S-NO group, 7.53 (95% CI, 4.01–14.14) in the NS-O group, and 11.59 (95% CI, 6.72–19.98) in the S-O group, compared with the NS-NO group. Although there is no evidence of a relationship of sarcopenic obesity with CVD events, sarcopenic obesity may be a risk for CVD via dyslipidemia, hypertension, and metabolic syndrome. These studies suggest that when assessing the impact of obesity on CVD, it may be important to assess the existence of sarcopenic obesity. However, the definition and gold standard for assessment of sarcopenic obesity have not yet been established, and further studies are therefore needed.

7.2 Diabetes Mellitus as a Risk Factor for Cardiovascular Disease in the Elderly

The epidemic of diabetes mellitus in the elderly is an important global problem as well as obesity. In Japan, the prevalence of diabetes mellitus increases with age, and prevalences of type 2 diabetes defined as HbA1c (NGSP) of 6.5% or more were

25% and 14% in men and women aged 60 years or over, respectively, based on the National Health and Nutrition Survey in 2015. A large-scale meta-regression analysis showed that a substantial increase in the prevalence of diabetes from 7.8% to 9.8% is expected in Japan during the next few decades, mainly as a result of aging of the adult population [13]. The proportion of individuals over 60 years of age who have diabetes mellitus is now more than two-thirds of the estimated total number of patients with diabetes mellitus in Japan. According to our cohort data, the prevalence of type 2 diabetes increased with age, and 48% of the individuals with type 2 diabetes who underwent health checkups were aged over 70 years. Decrease in both insulin secretion and action, decrease in muscle mass and relative increase in visceral fat, and decrease in insulin sensitivity with aging have been reported as mechanism of the deterioration in glucose tolerance in elderly people [14–17].

Elderly patients with type 2 diabetes are more likely than middle-aged patients to have diabetic microangiopathy and macroangiopathy. One of the reasons is that the duration of diabetes mellitus is likely to be longer in elderly patients than in the middle-aged patients. Another reason is that elderly patients frequently have several comorbidities such as hypertension and dyslipidemia, and accumulation of these risk factors accelerates the development of diabetic complications. Huang et al. reported the rates of complications in older patients with diabetes mellitus according to the results of the Diabetes and Aging Study [18]. The cohort study that included 72,310 older patients (≥60 years of age) with type 2 diabetes showed that the higher the age category was (60–69, 70–79, and ≥80 years of age), the higher were the incidences of atherosclerotic complications such as coronary artery disease, cerebrovascular disease, and congestive heart failure. In older adults with a shorter duration of type 2 diabetes (0–9 years), the incidences of coronary artery disease in the age group of 60–69, 70–79, and ≥80 years were 8.48, 11.47, and 15.09 (/1000 person-years), respectively; the incidences of cerebrovascular disease were 5.41, 9.83, and 17.79 (/1000 person-years), respectively; and the incidences of congestive heart failure were 6.82, 12.64, and 24.24 (/1000 person-years), respectively. In older adults with a longer duration of type 2 diabetes (≥10 years), similar relations of age categories with incidences of the above three cardiovascular events were observed, but all of the incidences were higher in the longer duration group than in the shorter duration group.

Kuusisto et al. reported that type 2 diabetes in the elderly was a strong risk factor for future occurrence of coronary heart disease (CHD) [19]. The results of their observational study that included 1298 elderly Finnish individuals (65–74 years of age) with a 3.5-year follow-up period showed that presence of hyperglycemia (HbA1c ≥ 7.0%) and duration of diabetes were significant risk factors for all CHD events or CHD death. The odds ratios of type 2 diabetes with HbA1c ≥7.0% hyperglycemia for CHD events and CHD death were 2.2 and 4.3, respectively.

Cardiovascular Prevention from Observational Cohorts in the Japan Research Group (EPOCH-JAPAN), which is a large-scale pooled analysis of Japanese community-based cohort studies including our cohort data, showed an age-specific association of diabetes with cardiovascular risk, especially in the elderly [20]. A total of 38,854 individuals (including 1867 individuals with diabetes mellitus) who had no history of CVD were registered from 8 cohorts, and the mean follow-up

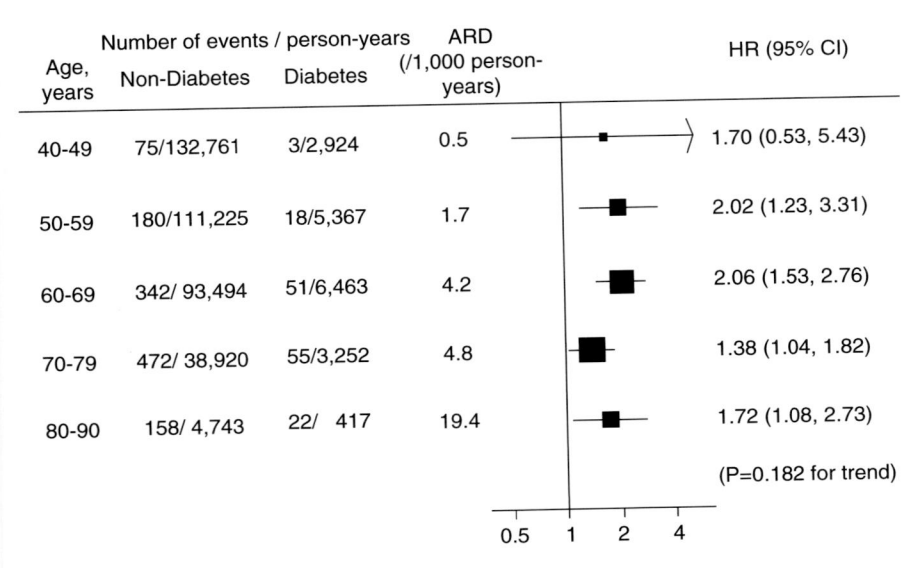

Fig. 7.3 Relative and absolute risks of death from cardiovascular disease associated with diabetes in each age group. The HRs and 95% CIs were calculated among age groups using the sex-adjusted stratified Cox model. The trend in the influence of diabetes on cardiovascular risk across age categories was tested by adding a multiplicative interaction term between diabetic status and ordinal age groups to the relevant Cox model.
HR hazard ratio, *CI* confidence interval, *ARD* absolute risk difference [20]

period was 10.3 years. The hazard ratios of diabetes mellitus for CVD death increased with age, and the hazard ratios in the age group of 40–49, 50–59, 60–69, 70–79, and 80–89 years were 1.70 (95% CI, 0.53–5.43), 2.02 (95% CI, 1.23–3.31), 2.06 (95% CI, 1.53–2.76), 1.38 (95% CI, 1.04–1.82), and 1.72 (95% CI, 1.08–2.73), respectively (Fig. 7.3).

Poorly controlled diabetes is one of the strong risk factors for CVD or all-cause death in the elderly population as well as in the middle-aged population [21]. However, several studies have shown that there is a J-curve phenomenon in the relationship between HbA1c and CVD events or all-cause mortality in elderly patients with type 2 diabetes. According to the results of the Japanese Elderly Diabetes Intervention Trial (J-EDIT) [22], which was a randomized control trial to evaluate the effects of multiple risk factor interventions on functional prognosis and development and on progression of diabetic complications and CVD in 1173 elderly type 2 diabetes patients (≥65 years of age) with a 6-year follow-up period, HbA1c and non-HDL cholesterol level were significant risk factors for stroke. The hazard ratios of HbA1c (/1%) and non-HDL cholesterol (/1 mg/dL) for stroke were 1.36 and 1.01, respectively. When participants were divided into quartile categories according to HbA1c level, the cumulative incidence of stroke was lowest in the second lowest quartile (HbA1c 7.3–7.9%), and the incidence was significantly higher in the highest quartile (≥8.8%) than in the second quartile. The relationship was J-shaped (Fig. 7.4).

Fig. 7.4 Glycated hemoglobin A1c (HbA1c) and incidence of stroke. The highest HbA1c quartile (38.8%) had an increased incidence of stroke compared with the second lowest (*P* = 0.003), second highest (*P* = 0.008), and lowest (*P* = 0.092) quartiles. The incidence of stroke was lowest in the second lowest HbA1c quartile (7.3–7.9%). This suggests the existence of a J-curve incidence of stroke according to the HbA1c distribution [22]

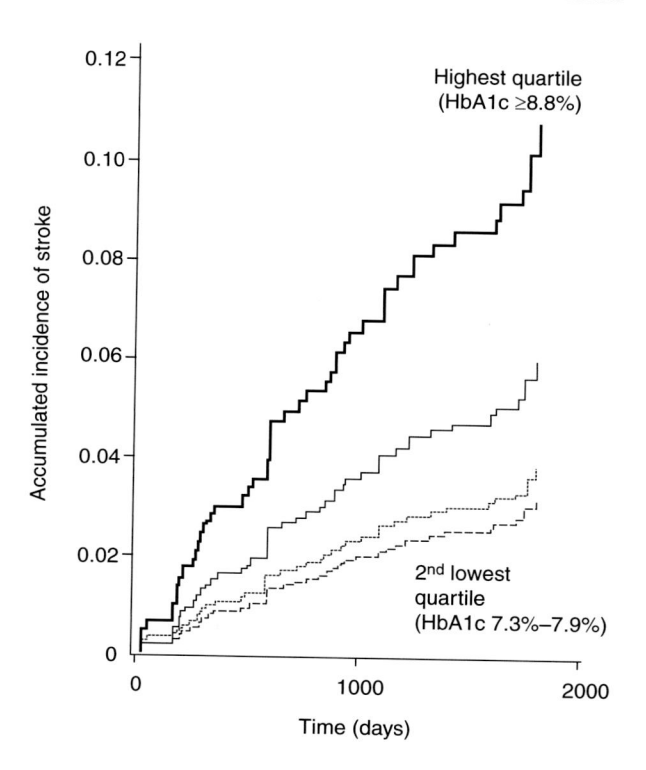

A similar relation was observed in the Diabetes and Aging Study, which included 71,092 older patients with type 2 diabetes [23]. The mean age of the population was 71.0 years, and mean HbA1c was 7.0%. The mean follow-up period was 3.1 years, and mortality was 40.4 per 1000 person-years. The participants were divided into seven groups according to HbA1c level at baseline: HbA1c of <6.0%, 6.0–6.9%, 7.0–7.9%, 8.0–8.9%, 9.0–9.9%, 10.0–10.9%, and ≥11.0%. The hazard ratios of HbA1c categories for all-cause mortality compared with the reference group (HbA1c of <6.0%) were 0.84 (95% CI, 0.79–0.90), 0.83 (95% CI, 0.76–0.90), 0.90 (95% CI, 0.81–1.00), 1.02 (95% CI, 0.88–1.17), 1.21 (95% CI, 1.01–1.45), and 1.31 (95% CI, 1.09–1.57) in the 6.0–6.9%, 7.0–7.9%, 8.0–8.9%, 9.0–9.9%, 10.0–10.9%, and ≥11.0% groups, respectively. The relationship was also J-curved in that analysis.

These J-curved relations suggest that intensive control of diabetes mellitus may be a risk of increase in stroke and mortality. Intensive control of diabetes mellitus causes severe hypoglycemia, and severe hypoglycemia may increase CVD events in elderly individuals with diabetes mellitus [24]. Severe hypoglycemia also leads to an increase in cognitive impairment in elderly patients [25]. It is necessary to achieve both maintenance of a good control level of blood glucose to avoid long-term complications and minimization of hypoglycemia- and hypoglycemia-associated morbidity and mortality.

References

1. Flegal KM, Carroll MD, Kit BK, Ogden CL. Prevalence of obesity and trends in the distribution of body mass index among US adults, 1999-2010. JAMA. 2012;307(5):491–7.
2. Han TS, Tajar A, Lean ME. Obesity and weight management in the elderly. Br Med Bull. 2011;97:169–96.
3. Ohnishi H, Saitoh S, Takagi S, Katoh N, Chiba Y, Akasaka H, et al. Incidence of type 2 diabetes in individuals with central obesity in a rural Japanese population: the Tanno and Sobetsu study. Diabetes Care. 2006;29(5):1128–9.
4. Ohnishi H, Saitoh S, Akasaka H, Mitsumata K, Chiba M, Furugen M, et al. Incidence of hypertension in individuals with abdominal obesity in a rural Japanese population: the Tanno and Sobetsu study. Hypertens Res. 2008;31(7):1385–90.
5. Fujii M, Ohnishi H, Saitho S, Mori M, Shimamoto K. Comparison of the effect of abdominal obesity on new onset of type 2 diabetes in a general Japanese elderly population with that in a non-elderly population-the Tanno and Sobetsu study. Nihon Ronen Igakkai Zasshi. Jpn J Geriatr. 2011;48(1):71–7.
6. Mitsumata K, Saitoh S, Ohnishi H, Akasaka H, Miura T. Effects of parental hypertension on longitudinal trends in blood pressure and plasma metabolic profile: mixed-effects model analysis. Hypertension. 2012;60(5):1124–30.
7. Saito I, Kokubo Y, Kiyohara Y, Doi Y, Saitoh S, Ohnishi H, et al. Prospective study on waist circumference and risk of all-cause and cardiovascular mortality: pooled analysis of Japanese community-based studies. Circ J. 2012;76(12):2867–74.
8. Hildrum B, Mykletun A, Dahl AA, Midthjell K. Metabolic syndrome and risk of mortality in middle-aged versus elderly individuals: the Nord-Trondelag Health Study (HUNT). Diabtologia. 2009;52(4):583–90.
9. Kohara K. Sarcopenic obesity in aging population: current status and future directions for research. Endocrine. 2014;45(1):15–25.
10. Baek SJ, Nam GE, Han KD, Choi SW, Jung SW, Bok AR, et al. Sarcopenia and sarcopenic obesity and their association with dyslipidemia in Korean elderly men: the 2008-2010 Korea National Health and Nutrition Examination Survey. J Endocrinol Investig. 2014;37(3):247–60.
11. Han K, Park YM, Kwon HS, Ko SH, Lee SH, Yim HW, et al. Sarcopenia as a determinant of blood pressure in older Koreans: findings from the Korea National Health and Nutrition Examination Surveys (KNHANES) 2008-2010. PLoS One. 2014;9(1):e86902.
12. Lu CW, Yang KC, Chang HH, Lee LT, Chen CY, Huang KC. Sarcopenic obesity is closely associated with metabolic syndrome. Obes Res Clin Pract. 2013;7(4):e301–7.
13. Charvat H, Goto A, Goto M, Inoue M, Heianza Y, Arase Y, et al. Impact of population aging on trends in diabetes prevalence: a meta-regression analysis of 160,000 Japanese adults. J Diabetes Invest. 2015;6(5):533–42.
14. Tamura Y, Izumiyama-Shimomura N, Kimbara Y, Nakamura K, Ishikawa N, Aida J, et al. Telomere attrition in beta and alpha cells with age. Age. 2016;38(3):61.
15. Basu R, Breda E, Oberg AL, Powell CC, Dalla Man C, Basu A, et al. Mechanisms of the age-associated deterioration in glucose tolerance: contribution of alterations in insulin secretion, action, and clearance. Diabetes. 2003;52(7):1738–48.
16. Sakurai T, Iimuro S, Araki A, Umegaki H, Ohashi Y, Yokono K, et al. Age-associated increase in abdominal obesity and insulin resistance, and usefulness of AHA/NHLBI definition of metabolic syndrome for predicting cardiovascular disease in Japanese elderly with type 2 diabetes mellitus. Gerontology. 2010;56(2):141–9.
17. Tamura Y, Izumiyama-Shimomura N, Kimbara Y, Nakamura K, Ishikawa N, Aida J, et al. beta-cell telomere attrition in diabetes: inverse correlation between HbA1c and telomere length. J Clin Endocrinol Metab. 2014;99(8):2771–7.

18. Huang ES, Laiteerapong N, Liu JY, John PM, Moffet HH, Karter AJ. Rates of complications and mortality in older patients with diabetes mellitus: the diabetes and aging study. JAMA Intern Med. 2014;174(2):251–8.
19. Kuusisto J, Mykkanen L, Pyorala K, Laakso M. NIDDM and its metabolic control predict coronary heart disease in elderly subjects. Diabetes. 1994;43(8):960–7.
20. Hirakawa Y, Ninomiya T, Kiyohara Y, Murakami Y, Saitoh S, Nakagawa H, et al. Age-specific impact of diabetes mellitus on the risk of cardiovascular mortality: an overview from the evidence for Cardiovascular Prevention from Observational Cohorts in the Japan Research Group (EPOCH-JAPAN). J Epidemiol. 2017;27(3):123–9.
21. van Hateren KJ, Landman GW, Kleefstra N, Drion I, Groenier KH, Houweling ST, et al. Glycaemic control and the risk of mortality in elderly type 2 diabetic patients (ZODIAC-20). Int J Clin Pract. 2011;65(4):415–9.
22. Araki A, Iimuro S, Sakurai T, Umegaki H, Iijima K, Nakano H, et al. Non-high-density lipoprotein cholesterol: an important predictor of stroke and diabetes-related mortality in Japanese elderly diabetic patients. Geriatr Gerontol Int. 2012;12(Suppl 1):18–28.
23. Huang ES, Liu JY, Moffet HH, John PM, Karter AJ. Glycemic control, complications, and death in older diabetic patients: the diabetes and aging study. Diabetes Care. 2011;34(6):1329–36.
24. Desouza CV, Bolli GB, Fonseca V. Hypoglycemia, diabetes, and cardiovascular events. Diabetes Care. 2010;33(6):1389–94.
25. Mattishent K, Loke YK. Bi-directional interaction between hypoglycaemia and cognitive impairment in elderly patients treated with glucose-lowering agents: a systematic review and meta-analysis. Diabetes Obes Metab. 2016;18(2):135–41.

Chapter 8
Blood Pressure and Cardiovascular Disease in the Elderly

Kei Asayama and Takayoshi Ohkubo

Abstract Even though Japan has the longest life expectancy in the world, blood pressure has not been adequately controlled, irrespective of age. More than half of Japanese individuals of ≥ 70 years of age had blood pressure levels of $\geq 140/\geq 90$ mmHg. Though the impact of blood pressure on cardiovascular complications differs according to the age, blood pressure lowering treatment reduces cardiovascular risk across various baseline blood pressure levels and comorbidities. Meanwhile, antihypertensive treatment itself is a sort of marker of the chronicity and severity of blood pressure elevation as well as the subclinical disease burden. Clinicians who initiate antihypertensive drug therapy should therefore recognize that patients have an increased risk in general, e.g., they fail to make lifestyle modifications, not just only related to their blood pressure level. Furthermore, self-measured home blood pressure is more reliable prognostic factors than the conventional office blood pressure, and affordable and validated automated devices for the self-measurement of home blood pressure are readily available. The careful and intensive follow-up of elderly individuals with hypertension is essential, and active utilization of the self-measured home blood pressure is desirable.

Keywords Blood pressure · Elderly · Cardiovascular disease · Out-of-office blood pressure · Self-measured home blood pressure · Antihypertensive drug therapy · Epidemiology · Population science · Clinical trial

K. Asayama (✉) · T. Ohkubo
Department of Hygiene and Public Health, Teikyo University School of Medicine, Tokyo, Japan

Tohoku Institute for Management of Blood Pressure, Sendai, Japan
e-mail: kei@asayama.org

8.1 Introduction

The impact of blood pressure on cardiovascular complications differs according to the age of the individual [1, 2]. Systolic blood pressure levels increase with age, while diastolic blood pressure values peak at approximately 60 years of age [3]; thus, isolated systolic hypertension, systolic blood pressure ≥140 mmHg with diastolic blood pressure <90 mmHg, is dominant among elderly individuals [4], and systolic blood pressure is a main driver of the risk of cardiovascular disease. In this section, we provide an overview of the current blood pressure level and the impact of blood pressure on cardiovascular complications in relation to antihypertensive drug treatment and blood pressure information, i.e., conventional office and out-of-office home blood pressure.

8.2 Blood Pressure and Its Control in Relation to Aging

Over the long term, an affluent lifestyle can influence the progression of arteriosclerosis. Because both environmental and genetic factors affect the blood pressure trend with age, standardized epidemiological methods that integrate clinical, environmental, and genetic information are necessary to clarify the natural course of blood pressure changes that occur in relation to aging.

The systolic blood pressure level generally increases with age [3]; in Japan, however, the systolic blood pressure levels have gradually decrease since 1965 [5–7]. The spontaneous increase that is observed in the systolic blood pressure with aging is not observed in the diastolic blood pressure. According to the Fifth National Survey on Circulatory Disorders in Japan [8] and the collaborative meta-analysis of individual participant data Japan Arteriosclerosis Longitudinal Study (JALS) [3], the ceiling of diastolic blood pressure in individuals without antihypertensive drug treatment is observed before 60 years of age in men and before 70 years of age in women (Fig. 8.1). Among patients who receive antihypertensive drug medication, an obvious inverse association between age and diastolic blood pressure was found, regardless of sex [3].

Even though Japan has the longest life expectancy in the world [9], blood pressure has not been adequately controlled, irrespective of age [3]. Several studies have reported that more than half of Japanese individuals of ≥70 years of age had blood pressure levels of ≥140/≥90 mmHg [3, 10, 11]. Approximately 1 million US residents in the Practice Innovation and Clinical Excellence (PINNACLE) clinical registry (white, 85.4%; black, 11.9%; antihypertensive drug nonusers, 26.3%) were assessed between 2008 and 2012. Among the patients with hypertension, 66.9% of the patients who were ≥60 years of age without diabetes fulfilled the treatment goal of <140/<90 mmHg [12]. For the prevention of cardiovascular disease in elderly individuals, we should routinely consider reducing their blood pressure to the normotensive range [13].

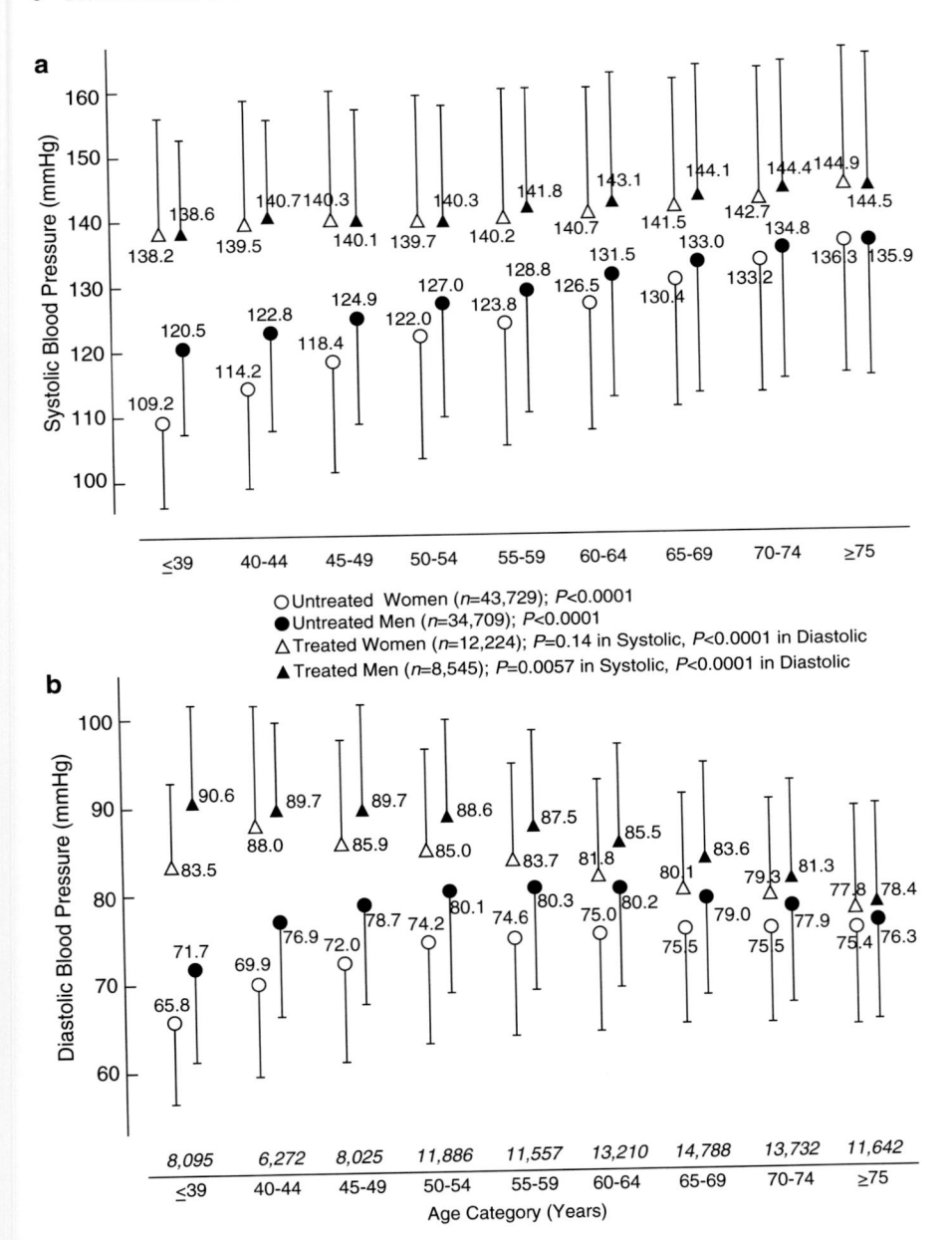

Fig. 8.1 The systolic (**a**) and diastolic (**b**) blood pressure according to age category and treatment status. Women and men without antihypertensive drug treatment at baseline are represented as open and filled circles, respectively. Those with treatment are represented as corresponding triangles. Vertical lines represent one side of the SD. Numbers on the horizontal axis indicate the number of participants in each age category. *P* values denote the linearity among age groups. Reproduced from Asayama and colleagues [3]

8.3 The Impact of Blood Pressure Reduction in Clinical Trials

Blood pressure lowering treatment reduces cardiovascular risk across various baseline blood pressure levels and comorbidities [13]. In a recent meta-analysis of 613,815 participants from 123 randomized trials, a 10-mmHg decrease in systolic blood pressure was associated with a significant 20% reduction (95% CI, 17–23%) in the incidence of major adverse cardiovascular events (MACE) [13]. However, there has not been a specific target blood pressure for treating hypertension in the elderly. In the Systolic Hypertension in the Elderly Program (SHEP) trial, which included patients of ≥60 years of age with systolic hypertension (systolic, ≥160 mmHg), antihypertensive drug treatment reduced the incidence of total stroke and MACE [14]. The Hypertension in the Very Elderly Trial (HYVET) demonstrated the benefit of active treatment in individuals of ≥80 years of age [15]. In contrast, the Japanese Trial to Assess Optimal Systolic Blood Pressure in Elderly Hypertensive Patients (JATOS) [16] and the Valsartan in Elderly Isolated Systolic Hypertension (VALISH) trial failed to identify any benefits of reducing the systolic blood pressure to <140 mmHg in elderly patients [16, 17]. This may be because these trials [16, 17] were underpowered; the observed event rate in VALISH was less than half the rate estimated in the protocol setting [17].

The Systolic Blood Pressure Intervention Trial (SPRINT) is a landmark study of the treatment of hypertension in both the general [18] and elderly [19] populations. The trial randomized 9631 patients of ≥50 years of age with moderate cardiovascular risk and a systolic blood pressure of 130–180 mmHg [18]. Patients with diabetes and those with history of a prior stroke were excluded because the same study group reported that intensive blood pressure reduction among such patients did not significantly reduce the rate of MACE, although a marginal reduction was observed (HR 0.88; 95% CI, 0.73–1.06) [20]. The research group compared a systolic blood pressure goal of <140 mmHg with a goal of <120 mmHg among 2636 hypertensive patients of ≥75 years of age in SPRINT. In comparison to the former standard treatment group, the latter intensive treatment group demonstrated a significantly greater reduction of MACE by 34% (95% CI, 15–49%), and a 33% (95% CI, 9–51%) reduction of all-cause mortality [19]. The absolute cardiovascular event rates in the subgroup of the approximately 30% of the patients who exhibited frailty were also lower in the intensive treatment group [19].

Different from SPRINT, among men of ≥55 years and women of ≥65 years who were classified as intermediate risk in the Heart Outcomes Prevention Evaluation (HOPE)-3 trial ($n = 12,705$), therapy with candesartan (16 mg/day) plus hydrochlorothiazide (12.5 mg/day) failed to reduce the incidence of MACE in comparison to a placebo (relative risk reduction, 7%; 95% CI, −10% to 21%) [21]. Besides advanced age, many possible reasons for the findings of SPRINT and HOPE-3, as well as other trials, were discussed [22, 23], including antihypertensive drug agents; for instance, chlorthalidone, which was used in SPRINT, has a greater preventive effect against cardiovascular complications than hydrochlorothiazide [22]. We should note that eligible patients who were allocated to the intensive treatment group in SPRINT showed a 14.8/7.6 mmHg reduction in blood pressure [18, 23]. In HOPE-3, participants in the active treatment group with a systolic blood pressure that was in the upper third (>143.5 mmHg; mean, 154.1 ± 8.9 mmHg) had nominally significantly lower rates of MACE in comparison to those in the placebo group (HR, 0.73; 95% CI, 0.56–0.94) [21, 23]. Based on the SPRINT findings [19] as well as the findings in this HOPE-3 subgroup [21], intensive blood pressure lowering treatment appears to be less harmful, at least among elderly patients with hypertension and moderate cardiovascular risk.

8.4 Recent Findings from the EPOCH-JAPAN Observational Study

The early introduction of antihypertensive medication has a long-term beneficial effect with regard to cardiovascular events [24]. However, people using antihypertensive medication were found to have a higher cardiovascular risk in comparison to those without treatment for a given level of baseline blood pressure after adjustment for major confounding factors [25–27]. Antihypertensive treatment itself is a sort of marker of the chronicity and severity of blood pressure elevation as well as the subclinical disease burden in observational studies [25–28]. The most important explanation for treated hypertensive patients who still have a high cardiovascular risk is lack of control of blood pressure and of other risk factors [28]. Not just related to the blood pressure level alone, clinicians who initiate antihypertensive drug therapy should recognize that patients have an increased risk in general, e.g., they fail to make lifestyle modifications [29].

To clarify the impact of antihypertensive drug treatment on the blood pressure level and the residual cardiovascular risk in elderly population, an individual-level meta-analysis was conducted among 26,133 participants of 60–89 years of age who were recruited from 1980 to 1995 from seven general population cohorts and who were enrolled in the Evidence for Cardiovascular Prevention from Observational Cohorts in Japan (EPOCH-JAPAN) [30]. Participants were cross-classified by age category, 60–74 years (young-old) versus 75–89 years (old-old), and by the usage of antihypertensive medication at baseline. Individual blood pressure levels were categorized into six categories according to the recent hypertension guidelines [31, 32]. Among the 4150 old-old participants, 32.2% received antihypertensive medication at baseline. The blood pressures of the treated participants, in reference to the risk for the untreated population, were 12.3 (95% CI, 11.7–12.9)/5.5 (5.2–5.9) mmHg higher among the young-old and 7.6 (6.2–9.1)/2.4 (1.6–3.2) mmHg higher among the old-old. The risk of cardiovascular mortality among the treated participants compared with the untreated population was consistently higher in the young-old (HR, 1.30; 95% CI, 1.16–1.46) and old-old participants (HR, 1.35; 95% CI, 1.16–1.56).

In the EPOCH-JAPAN database, the risks of cardiovascular mortality in the six blood pressure categories according to the treatment status are shown in Fig. 8.2. Irrespective of the antihypertensive medication status, the increase in the risk of total cardiovascular mortality that occurred with the elevation of blood pressure was significant among the young-old ($P \leq 0.0008$), but not significant among old-old

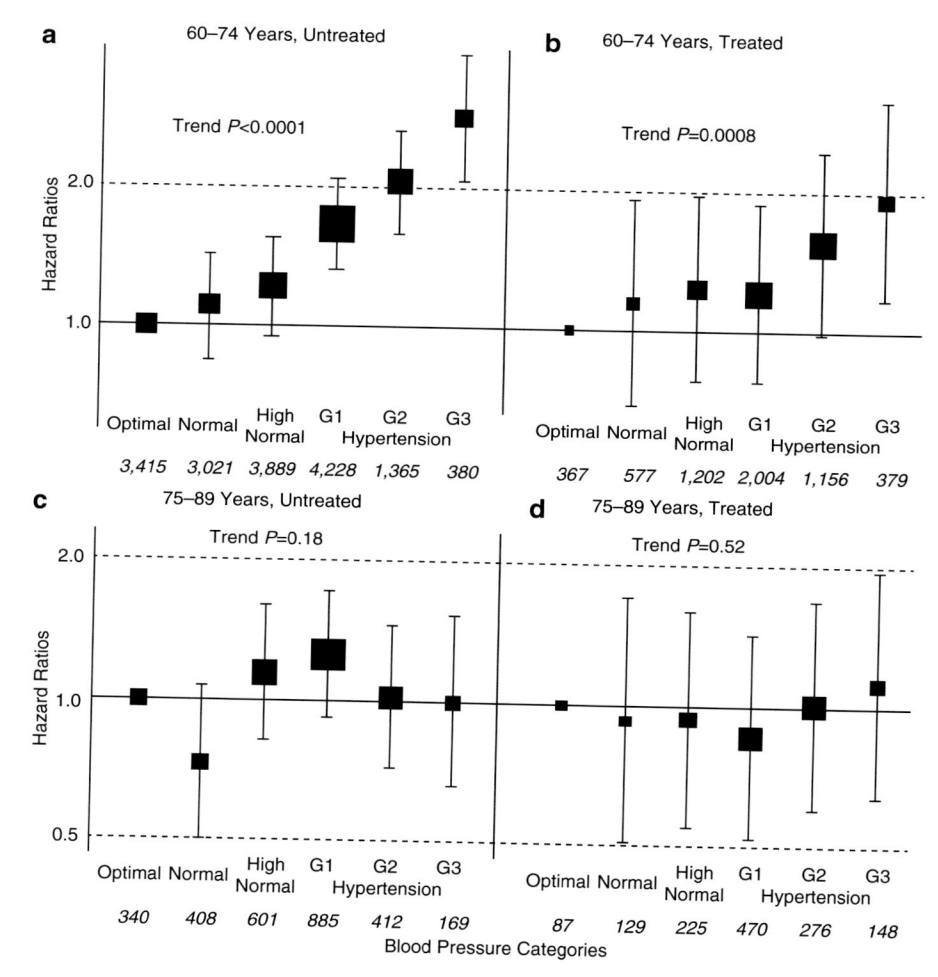

Fig. 8.2 The risk of total cardiovascular mortality among six blood pressure levels in untreated (**a, c**) and treated (**b, d**) participants of 60–74 years of age (**a, b**) and 75–89 years of age (**c, d**). Filled squares represent the hazard ratios in comparison to an optimal blood pressure level and are sized in proportion to the number of total cardiovascular deaths observed. Vertical bars indicate the 95% confidence intervals at each level. Blood pressure levels are defined as optimal (<120/<80 mmHg), normal (120–129/80–84 mmHg), high normal (130–139/85–89 mmHg), grade 1 (G1) hypertension (140–159/90–99 mmHg), grade 2 (G2) hypertension (160–179/100–109 mmHg), and grade 3 (G3) hypertension (≥180/≥110 mmHg). Trend P values denote the linearity among the six blood pressure levels. Adjustment was performed for sex, age, body mass index, history of cardiovascular disease, total cholesterol, lipid-lowering medication, diabetes mellitus, smoking, habitual drinking, and cohort. Reproduced from Asayama and colleagues [25]

participants ($P \geq 0.18$). The importance of blood pressure control in the elderly should not be underestimated [14, 19, 33, 34]; however, the precautions related to antihypertensive drug therapy in the elderly population vary. Chronological age alone is not sufficient for making useful judgments in relation to therapy [35], and the application of antihypertensive drug therapy should be based on factors that reflect the individual's condition, e.g., frailty and the cognitive function. Because the impact of blood pressure and the benefit of treatment are expected to be lower in older individuals [36], the early detection of hypertension and prompt intervention, including lifestyle modifications [37], is crucial to the long-term approach. Furthermore, we should be vigilant to detect residual cardiovascular risks in treated elderly hypertensive patients [26, 28], despite the fact that these risks are not well specified.

8.5 Out-of-Office Blood Pressure: Self-Measurement at Home

Out-of-office blood pressure, the self-measured home blood pressure and ambulatory blood pressure monitoring, is more reliable prognostic factors than the conventional office blood pressure, which is measured in an outpatient clinic or a health check center [38]. The superiority of out-of-office blood pressure over conventional blood pressure for the prediction of cardiovascular events also applies to older patients in general practice [39]. In the Systolic Hypertension in Europe (Syst-Eur) trial, the ambulatory systolic blood pressure was found to be a significant predictor of the cardiovascular risk among untreated elderly with isolated systolic hypertension and was superior to the conventional blood pressure in this regard [40]. The exclusive use of conventional blood pressure would result in failure to recognize white-coat, which should be carefully monitored [41–43], and masked hypertension, which should be considered to be associated with a similar degree of risk to sustained hypertension [42].

Only a few studies have assessed the risk in relation to home blood pressure in octogenarians. The Predictive Values of Blood Pressure and Arterial Stiffness in Institutionalized Very Aged Population Study (PARTAGE) [44, 45] included 1127 frail nursing home residents. Among these residents, 227 took ≥ 2 antihypertensive drugs with a systolic home blood pressure of <130 mmHg (averaged 119/65 mmHg). The mortality rates in these residents and the other 900 residents (averaged 142/75 mmHg) were 32.2% and 19.7%, respectively, and the adjusted HR for cardiovascular events associated with a low blood pressure with combination drug treatment was 1.28 (95% CI, 0.99–1.65) [44]. Moreover, in another analysis of the same cohort, the patients with a lower home diastolic blood pressure (49.3–68.5 mmHg) lived 2 years less than those with higher blood pressure ($P = 0.021$) [45]. These findings raise a cautionary note regarding the safety of combination drug therapy in frail elderly patients with a low systolic home blood pressure [46].

The International Database of HOme blood pressure in relation to Cardiovascular Outcome (IDHOCO) is a collaborating research project. In this project, an individual participant-level database was constructed and maintained at the Studies Coordinating Centre in Leuven, Belgium [47]. Three-hundred seventy-five octogenarians were enrolled in the IDHOCO [48]. A multivariable-adjusted Cox model revealed that among 202 untreated octogenarians, the risk of systolic home blood pressure reached statistical significance in the top fifth ($\geq$152.4 mmHg) for cardiovascular mortality (HR, 2.19; 95% CI, 1.04–4.64) and for all fatal plus nonfatal cardiovascular events combined (HR, 2.09; 95% CI, 1.11–3.91). In contrast, the HRs in the lower fifth ($\leq$65.1 mmHg) were significantly high ($P \leq 0.022$) while that in the upper fifth was significantly low for cardiovascular mortality ($P = 0.034$). The 5-year risk of a cardiovascular event showed an opposite trend between systolic and diastolic home blood pressure (Fig. 8.3). Whereas, among the other 173 octogenarians who were treated with antihypertensive medication at baseline, the relationship between cardiovascular events and the systolic blood pressure was curvilinear, independent of the diastolic blood pressure level, with a nadir at $\approx$150 mmHg, as shown in Fig. 8.4. Notwithstanding the potential limitations, the IDHOCO findings [48] have a number of implications for clinical practice: (1) a home diastolic blood pressure of <65 mmHg was associated with a worse cardiovascular prognosis, while values above $\approx$80 mmHg predicted a better outcome in untreated individuals, and (2) a systolic home blood pressure of <126.9 mmHg was associated with increased total mortality with the lowest risk at 148.6 mmHg in treated patients.

Recently, day-to-day home blood pressure variability is considered to be a risk factor for the development of dementia [49] (see Chap. 6) and cognitive decline [50].

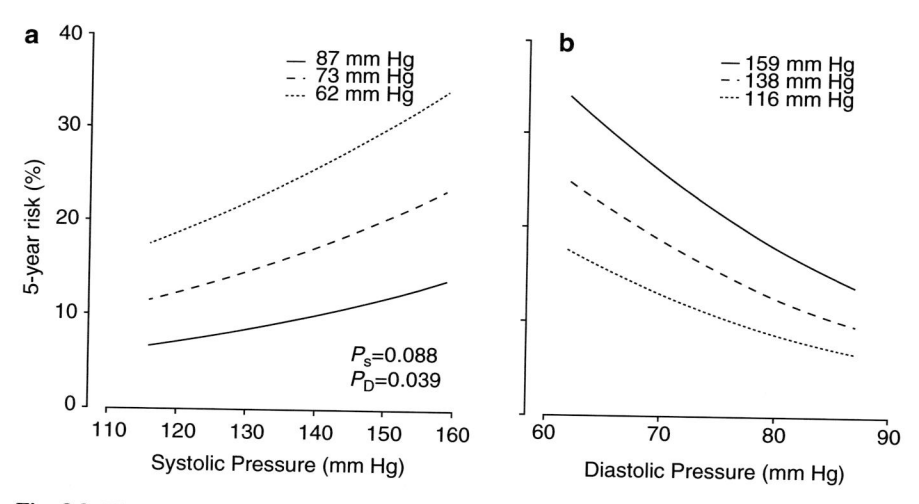

Fig. 8.3 The 5-year risk of a cardiovascular event associated with systolic (**a**) or diastolic (**b**) home blood pressure analyzed as continuous variables and across percentiles (10th, 50th, and 90th) of the alternative component of blood pressure in 202 untreated octogenarians. The risk was standardized according to the distribution (ratio or mean) in the whole untreated population of cohort, sex, age, body mass index, smoking and drinking, serum cholesterol, and history of cardiovascular disease and diabetes mellitus. P_S and P_D indicate the significance of the association with systolic and diastolic home blood pressure, respectively. Reproduced from Aparicio and colleagues [48]

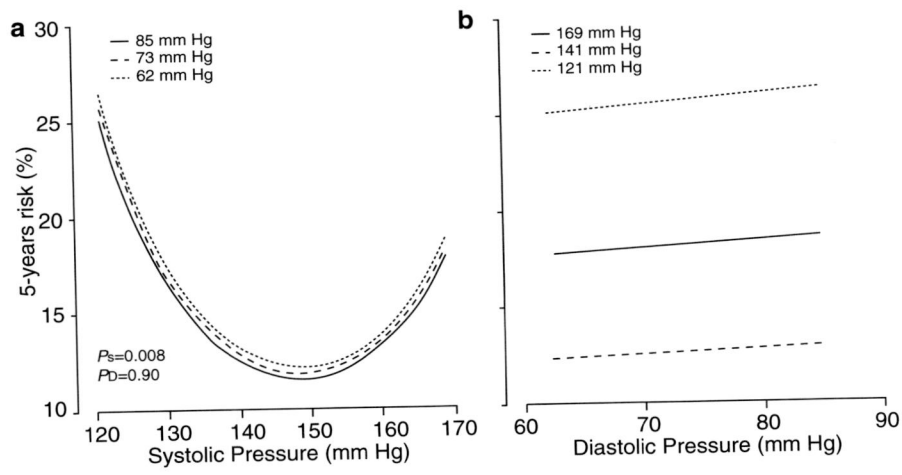

Fig. 8.4 The 5-year risk of a cardiovascular event associated with systolic (**a**) or diastolic (**b**) home blood pressure analyzed as continuous variables and across percentiles (10th, 50th, and 90th) of the alternative component of blood pressure in 173 treated octogenarians. The risk was standardized according to the distribution (ratio or mean) in the whole treated population of cohort, sex, age, body mass index, smoking and drinking, serum cholesterol, and history of cardiovascular disease and diabetes mellitus. P_S and P_D indicate the significance of the association with systolic and diastolic home blood pressure, respectively. The relationship with systolic blood pressure was U-shaped with a nadir at 148.6 mmHg. Reproduced from Aparicio and colleagues [48]

Among residents who participated in the Ohasama study, the home systolic blood pressure at baseline was significantly associated with cognitive decline after a median 7.8 years of follow-up (odds ratio per 1-SD increase, 1.48; $P = 0.03$); however, the conventional systolic blood pressure was not (odds ratio, 1.24; $P = 0.2$) [50]. Furthermore, the day-to-day variability in systolic blood pressure, represented as the SD, showed a significant association with cognitive decline after adjustment for the home systolic blood pressure level (odds ratio, 1.51; $P = 0.02$) [50]. Although the impact of the blood pressure level on cardiovascular complications is attenuated in old-old individuals in comparison to young-old and younger individuals [25, 30], we should pay careful attention to the other outcomes in these populations, and home blood pressure variability as well as the home blood pressure level may be a useful predictor of worse outcomes in the elderly population; however, it should be noted that home blood pressure variability would be difficult to be modified by drug treatment [51].

8.6 Perspectives

SPRINT demonstrated that antihypertensive drug treatment has a beneficial effect with regard to reducing cardiovascular complications in elderly patients with hypertension [52]. The optimal systolic blood pressure goal of <140 mmHg seems reasonable [4], and a more intensive treatment goal, e.g., <130/<80 mmHg for moderate- to high-risk old-old patients, can be recommended [52, 53]. Nevertheless, we should be cautious about the fact that patients on antihypertensive drug treatment had a 1.2–1.5-fold higher risk of cardiovascular mortality in comparison to untreated individuals [30] and that the impact of the blood pressure level decreases with age [30]. Patients with frequent falls, advanced cognitive impairment, and multiple comorbidities may be at risk of adverse outcomes with intensive blood pressure lowering, particularly under combination drug therapy [46], because such residents typically reside in nursing homes, require assistance for their daily living, and are never represented in modern randomized trials [53]. Once a patient starts antihypertensive drug treatment, the self-measurement of the home blood pressure should be performed for the long-term management of hypertension because the recording of the daily home measurements enables us to safely and conveniently monitor adverse effects. Home blood pressure measurement is feasible and can be largely diffused to the elderly individuals in the general population [54]. Furthermore, affordable and validated automated devices for the self-measurement of home blood pressure are readily available. The careful and intensive follow-up of elderly individuals with hypertension is essential [30], and active utilization of the self-measured home blood pressure is desirable.

Acknowledgments We gratefully acknowledge the secretary of the Department of Hygiene and Public Health, Teikyo University School of Medicine for their valuable support.

Sources of Funding None.

Conflict of Interests K. Asayama and T. Ohkubo are consultants for Omron Healthcare Co., Ltd (Kyoto, Japan).

References

1. Lewington S, Clarke R, Qizilbash N, Peto R, Collins R. Age-specific relevance of usual blood pressure to vascular mortality: a meta-analysis of individual data for one million adults in 61 prospective studies. Lancet. 2002;360(9349):1903–13.
2. Lawes CM, Rodgers A, Bennett DA, Parag V, Suh I, Ueshima H, et al. Blood pressure and cardiovascular disease in the Asia Pacific region. J Hypertens. 2003;21(4):707–16.
3. Asayama K, Hozawa A, Taguri M, Ohkubo T, Tabara Y, Suzuki K, et al. Blood pressure, heart rate, and double product in a pooled cohort: the Japan arteriosclerosis longitudinal study. J Hypertens. 2017;35(9):1808–15.
4. Bavishi C, Goel S, Messerli FH. Isolated systolic hypertension: an update after SPRINT. Am J Med. 2016;129(12):1251–8.
5. Miura K, Nagai M, Ohkubo T. Epidemiology of hypertension in Japan. Circ J. 2013; 77(9):2226–31.
6. Ueshima H. Explanation for the Japanese paradox: prevention of increase in coronary heart disease and reduction in stroke. J Atheroscler Thromb. 2007;14(6):278–86.
7. Ueshima H, Tatara K, Asakura S, Okamoto M. Declining trends in blood pressure level and the prevalence of hypertension, and changes in related factors in Japan, 1956–1980. J Chronic Dis. 1987;40(2):137–47.

8. Ministry of Health, Labor and Welfare. National survey on circulatory disease, 2000. Tokyo: Ministry of Health, Labor and Welfare; 2002.

9. World Health Organization. World Health Statistics 2016: Monitoring health for the SDGs. 2016. http://www.who.int/gho/publications/world_health_statistics/2016/en/.

10. Hozawa A, Ohkubo T, Kikuya M, Yamaguchi J, Ohmori K, Fujiwara T, et al. Blood pressure control assessed by home, ambulatory and conventional blood pressure measurements in the Japanese general population: the Ohasama study. Hypertens Res. 2002;25(1):57–63.

11. Ohkubo T, Obara T, Funahashi J, Kikuya M, Asayama K, Metoki H, et al. Control of blood pressure as measured at home and office, and comparison with physicians' assessment of control among treated hypertensive patients in Japan: first report of the Japan Home versus Office Blood Pressure Measurement Evaluation (J-HOME) study. Hypertens Res. 2004;27(10):755–63.

12. Borden WB, Maddox TM, Tang F, Rumsfeld JS, Oetgen WJ, Mullen JB, et al. Impact of the 2014 expert panel recommendations for management of high blood pressure on contemporary cardiovascular practice: insights from the NCDR PINNACLE registry. J Am Coll Cardiol. 2014;64(21):2196–203.

13. Ettehad D, Emdin CA, Kiran A, Anderson SG, Callender T, Emberson J, et al. Blood pressure lowering for prevention of cardiovascular disease and death: a systematic review and meta-analysis. Lancet. 2016;387(10022):957–67.

14. Prevention of stroke by antihypertensive drug treatment in older persons with isolated systolic hypertension. Final results of the Systolic Hypertension in the Elderly Program (SHEP). SHEP Cooperative Research Group. JAMA. 1991;265(24):3255–64.

15. Beckett NS, Peters R, Fletcher AE, Staessen JA, Liu L, Dumitrascu D, et al. Treatment of hypertension in patients 80 years of age or older. N Engl J Med. 2008;358(18):1887–98.

16. JATOS Study Group. Principal results of the Japanese trial to assess optimal systolic blood pressure in elderly hypertensive patients (JATOS). Hypertens Res. 2008;31(12):2115–27.

17. Ogihara T, Saruta T, Rakugi H, Matsuoka H, Shimamoto K, Shimada K, et al. Target blood pressure for treatment of isolated systolic hypertension in the elderly: valsartan in elderly isolated systolic hypertension study. Hypertension. 2010;56(2):196–202.

18. SPRINT Research Group, Wright JT Jr, Williamson JD, Whelton PK, Snyder JK, Sink KM, et al. A randomized trial of intensive versus standard blood-pressure control. N Engl J Med. 2015;373(22):2103–16.

19. Williamson JD, Supiano MA, Applegate WB, Berlowitz DR, Campbell RC, Chertow GM, et al. Intensive vs standard blood pressure control and cardiovascular disease outcomes in adults aged >/=75 years: a randomized clinical trial. JAMA. 2016;315(24):2673–82.

20. Cushman WC, Evans GW, Byington RP, Goff DC Jr, Grimm RH Jr, Cutler JA, et al. Effects of intensive blood-pressure control in type 2 diabetes mellitus. N Engl J Med. 2010;362(17):1575–85.

21. Lonn EM, Bosch J, Lopez-Jaramillo P, Zhu J, Liu L, Pais P, et al. Blood-pressure lowering in intermediate-risk persons without cardiovascular disease. N Engl J Med. 2016;374(21):2009–20.

22. Whelton PK, Reboussin DM, Fine LJ. Comparing the SPRINT and the HOPE-3 blood pressure trial. JAMA Cardiol. 2016;1(8):855–6.

23. Yusuf S, Lonn E. The SPRINT and the HOPE-3 trial in the context of other blood pressure-lowering trials. JAMA Cardiol. 2016;1(8):857–8.

24. Bosch J, Lonn E, Pogue J, Arnold JM, Dagenais GR, Yusuf S, et al. Long-term effects of ramipril on cardiovascular events and on diabetes: results of the HOPE study extension. Circulation. 2005;112(9):1339–46.

25. Asayama K, Satoh M, Murakami Y, Ohkubo T, Nagasawa SY, Tsuji I, et al. Cardiovascular risk with and without antihypertensive drug treatment in the Japanese general population: participant-level meta-analysis. Hypertension. 2014;63(6):1189–97.

26. Asayama K, Ohkubo T, Yoshida S, Suzuki K, Metoki H, Harada A, et al. Stroke risk and antihypertensive drug treatment in the general population: the Japan arteriosclerosis longitudinal study. J Hypertens. 2009;27(2):357–64.

27. Lieb W, Enserro DM, Sullivan LM, Vasan RS. Residual cardiovascular risk in individuals on blood pressure-lowering treatment. J Am Heart Assoc. 2015;4(11):e002155.
28. Ibsen H. Antihypertensive treatment and risk of cardiovascular complications: is the cure worse than the disease? J Hypertens. 2009;27(2):221–3.
29. Kjeldsen SE, Jamerson KA, Bakris GL, Pitt B, Dahlof B, Velazquez EJ, et al. Predictors of blood pressure response to intensified and fixed combination treatment of hypertension: the ACCOMPLISH study. Blood Press. 2008;17(1):7–17.
30. Asayama K, Ohkubo T, Satoh A, Tanaka S, Higashiyama A, Murakami Y, et al. Cardiovascular risk and blood pressure lowering treatment among elderly individuals: evidence for cardiovascular prevention from observational cohorts in Japan. J Hypertens. 2018;36:410–8.
31. Ogihara T, Kikuchi K, Matsuoka H, Fujita T, Higaki J, Horiuchi M, et al. The Japanese Society of Hypertension guidelines for the management of hypertension (JSH 2009). Hypertens Res. 2009;32(1):3–107.
32. Mancia G, Fagard R, Narkiewicz K, Redon J, Zanchetti A, Bohm M, et al. 2013 ESH/ESC guidelines for the management of arterial hypertension: the Task Force for the Management of Arterial Hypertension of the European Society of Hypertension (ESH) and of the European Society of Cardiology (ESC). Eur Heart J. 2013;34(28):2159–219.
33. Staessen JA, Wang JG, Thijs L. Cardiovascular protection and blood pressure reduction: a meta-analysis. Lancet. 2001;358(9290):1305–15.
34. Turnbull F. Effects of different blood-pressure-lowering regimens on major cardiovascular events: results of prospectively-designed overviews of randomised trials. Lancet. 2003;362(9395):1527–35.
35. Materson BJ, Garcia-Estrada M, Preston RA. Hypertension in the frail elderly. J Am Soc Hypertens. 2016;10(6):536–41.
36. Staessen JA, Fagard R, Thijs L, Celis H, Birkenhager WH, Bulpitt CJ, et al. Subgroup and per-protocol analysis of the randomized European Trial on Isolated Systolic Hypertension in the Elderly. Arch Intern Med. 1998;158(15):1681–91.
37. Shimamoto K, Ando K, Fujita T, Hasebe N, Higaki J, Horiuchi M, et al. The Japanese Society of Hypertension guidelines for the management of hypertension (JSH 2014). Hypertens Res. 2014;37(4):253–390.
38. Asayama K, Brguljan-Hitij J, Imai Y. Out-of-office blood pressure improves risk stratification in normotension and prehypertension people. Curr Hypertens Rep. 2014;16(10):478.
39. Fagard RH, Van Den Broeke C, De Cort P. Prognostic significance of blood pressure measured in the office, at home and during ambulatory monitoring in older patients in general practice. J Hum Hypertens. 2005;19(10):801–7.
40. Staessen JA, Thijs L, Fagard R, O'Brien ET, Clement D, de Leeuw PW, et al. Predicting cardiovascular risk using conventional vs ambulatory blood pressure in older patients with systolic hypertension. Systolic Hypertension in Europe Trial Investigators. JAMA. 1999;282(6):539–46.
41. Franklin SS, Thijs L, Hansen TW, Li Y, Boggia J, Kikuya M, et al. Significance of white-coat hypertension in older persons with isolated systolic hypertension: a meta-analysis using the International Database on Ambulatory Blood Pressure Monitoring in Relation to Cardiovascular Outcomes population. Hypertension. 2012;59(3):564–71.
42. Asayama K, Thijs L, Li Y, Gu YM, Hara A, Liu YP, et al. Setting thresholds to varying blood pressure monitoring intervals differentially affects risk estimates associated with white-coat and masked hypertension in the population. Hypertension. 2014;64(5):935–42.
43. Ugajin T, Hozawa A, Ohkubo T, Asayama K, Kikuya M, Obara T, et al. White-coat hypertension as a risk factor for the development of home hypertension: the Ohasama study. Arch Intern Med. 2005;165(13):1541–6.
44. Benetos A, Labat C, Rossignol P, Fay R, Rolland Y, Valbusa F, et al. Treatment with multiple blood pressure medications, achieved blood pressure, and mortality in older nursing home residents: the PARTAGE study. JAMA Intern Med. 2015;175(6):989–95.

45. Benetos A, Gautier S, Labat C, Salvi P, Valbusa F, Marino F, et al. Mortality and cardiovascular events are best predicted by low central/peripheral pulse pressure amplification but not by high blood pressure levels in elderly nursing home subjects: the PARTAGE (predictive values of blood pressure and arterial stiffness in institutionalized very aged population) study. J Am Coll Cardiol. 2012;60(16):1503–11.
46. Aronow WS. Multiple blood pressure medications and mortality among elderly individuals. JAMA. 2015;313(13):1362–3.
47. Niiranen TJ, Thijs L, Asayama K, Johansson JK, Ohkubo T, Kikuya M, et al. The International Database of HOme blood pressure in relation to Cardiovascular Outcome (IDHOCO): moving from baseline characteristics to research perspectives. Hypertens Res. 2012;35(11):1072–9.
48. Aparicio LS, Thijs L, Boggia J, Jacobs L, Barochiner J, Odili AN, et al. Defining thresholds for home blood pressure monitoring in octogenarians. Hypertension. 2015;66(4):865–73.
49. Oishi E, Ohara T, Sakata S, Fukuhara M, Hata J, Yoshida D, et al. Day-to-day blood pressure variability and risk of dementia in a general Japanese Elderly Population: the Hisayama study. Circulation. 2017;136(6):516–25.
50. Matsumoto A, Satoh M, Kikuya M, Ohkubo T, Hirano M, Inoue R, et al. Day-to-day variability in home blood pressure is associated with cognitive decline: the Ohasama study. Hypertension. 2014;63(6):1333–8.
51. Asayama K, Ohkubo T, Hanazawa T, Watabe D, Hosaka M, Satoh M, et al. Does antihypertensive drug class affect day-to-day variability of self-measured home blood pressure? The HOMED-BP study. J Am Heart Assoc. 2016;5(3):e002995.
52. Rochlani Y, Khan MH, Aronow WS. Managing hypertension in patients aged 75 years and older. Curr Hypertens Rep. 2017;19(11):88.
53. Whelton PK, Carey RM, Aronow WS, Casey DE Jr, Collins KJ, Dennison Himmelfarb C, et al. ACC/AHA/AAPA/ABC/ACPM/AGS/APhA/ASH/ASPC/NMA/PCNA guideline for the prevention, detection, evaluation, and management of high blood pressure in adults: a report of the American College of Cardiology/American Heart Association Task Force on Clinical Practice Guidelines. Hypertension. 2018;71(6):e13–e115..
54. Cacciolati C, Tzourio C, Dufouil C, Alperovitch A, Hanon O. Feasibility of home blood pressure measurement in elderly individuals: cross-sectional analysis of a population-based sample. Am J Hypertens. 2012;25(12):1279–85.

Chapter 9
Stroke in the Elderly Population

Masahiro Kamouchi

Abstract Stroke incidence and mortality increase with advancing age. Age is a nonmodifiable risk factor for stroke. Moreover, cardiovascular risk factors, such as hypertension, diabetes mellitus, dyslipidemia, and atrial fibrillation, are more prevalent in older people than in younger ones. Poststroke neurological deficits often impair activities of daily living in stroke patients; thus, stroke is a main cause of disability worldwide. Effective and efficient measures against stroke are urgently required, especially in aging societies, to prolong the healthy life expectancy of the population. Recent epidemiological studies and clinical trials have accumulated evidence regarding the effects of preventive treatment against stroke in the elderly population, as well as the risks and benefits of stroke treatment in older patients. However, there remain a number of issues regarding how to reduce the stroke incidence among elderly populations and improve clinical outcomes after stroke without increasing adverse events in elderly patients. In this chapter, we will discuss the current understanding of risk factor management to prevent stroke and the optimal treatment for stroke in the elderly population.

Keywords Risk factor · Stroke prevention · Stroke care · Older adults

Stroke is one of the leading causes of death and disability globally. The incidence of stroke increases with advancing age; therefore, stroke is a major health problem, especially in an aging society. Poststroke disability often impairs not only activities of daily living but also quality of life in patients. The reduction of stroke incidence and mortality and the alleviation of poststroke symptoms are critical issues to reduce the burden of stroke and prolong healthy life expectancy worldwide.

M. Kamouchi
Department of Health Care Administration and Management, Graduate School of Medical Sciences, Kyushu University, Fukuoka, Japan
e-mail: kamouchi@hcam.med.kyushu-u.ac.jp

© Springer Nature Singapore Pte Ltd. 2019
M. Washio, C. Kiyohara (eds.), *Health Issues and Care System for the Elderly*,
Current Topics in Environmental Health and Preventive Medicine,
https://doi.org/10.1007/978-981-13-1762-0_9

9.1 Epidemiology

9.1.1 Stroke Incidence

Age is a nonmodifiable but significant risk factor for stroke (Fig. 9.1). The incidence of ischemic and hemorrhagic stroke increases with age in men and women, irrespective of ethnic origin. However, the trends in age-specific incidence of stroke differ according to stroke subtypes and region or country. In the Hisayama study, which began in 1961 and established five cohorts consisting of residents in a Japanese community aged ≥40 years, stroke incidence consistently decreased, even in the elderly group [1]. However, the incidence rate of brain hemorrhage continuously increased over time in participants aged ≥80 years, although that of ischemic stroke decreased [2]. The Global Burden of Disease Study 2010 estimated regional and country-specific incidence of stroke in 1990, 2005, and 2010 [3]. In the past two decades, the incidence of ischemic stroke among people aged ≥75 years decreased in high-income countries but not in low-income counties. Incidence of hemorrhagic stroke decreased in both high- and low-income countries, whereas the incidence rates among people aged 20–64 years significantly increased in low- and middle-income countries [3].

Older patients with stroke are at high risk for recurrent stroke. We previously developed risk scores for stroke recurrence in Japanese patients with ischemic stroke, and age was identified as a factor in the score [4]. Similarly, the risk of stroke

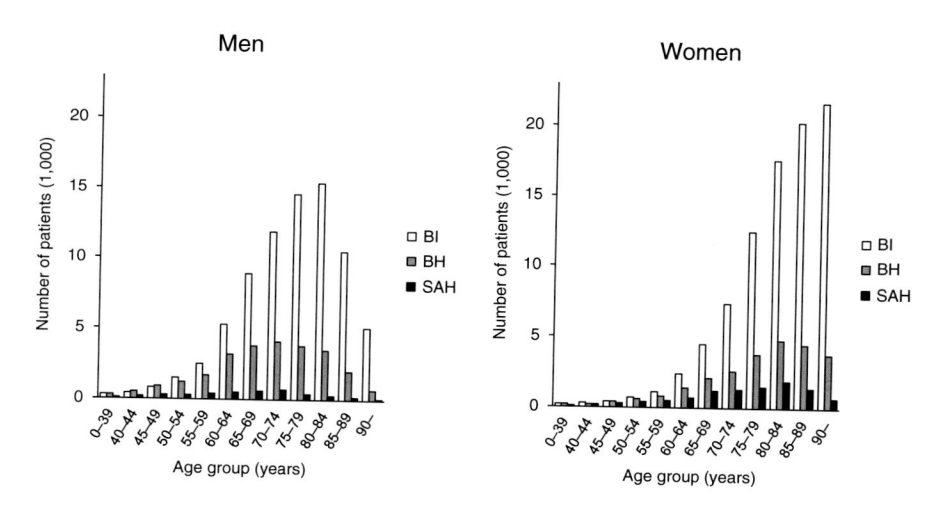

Fig. 9.1 Estimated number of patients with stroke in Japan, according to age. Estimated number of patients (inpatients and outpatients) with brain infarction (BI, white bars), brain hemorrhage (BH, shaded bars), and subarachnoid hemorrhage (SAH, black bars), shown according to each age group for men and women (Patient Survey 2014, Ministry of Health, Labour and Welfare)

after transient ischemic attack (TIA) increases with advancing age. In patients with TIA, age is a significant factor comprising risk scores to predict future stroke, such as ABCD score [5], ABCD2 score [6], and other related scores [7].

9.1.2 Stroke Mortality

Stroke mortality is declining in all countries [3, 8]. Nevertheless, stroke mortality remains high in people aged ≥75 years (Fig. 9.2). In high-income countries, age-standardized mortality rates have significantly decreased by a similar proportion in both younger and older people. However, in low- and middle-income countries, the reduction was less striking in people >75 years compared with younger people [8].

Case fatalities among stroke patients increase with advancing age. Among the Get With the Guidelines-Stroke population in the United States, the in-hospital case fatality was more than threefold higher in participants ≥80 years of age (10.3%) compared with those aged <50 years (3.0%) [9]. The adjusted odds ratio for in-hospital mortality has been reported as 1.27 (95% confidence interval [CI] 1.25–1.29) per 10-year increase [10]. Between 1990 and 2010, mortality-to-incidence rates were reduced in people <75 years compared with older people across all countries [8].

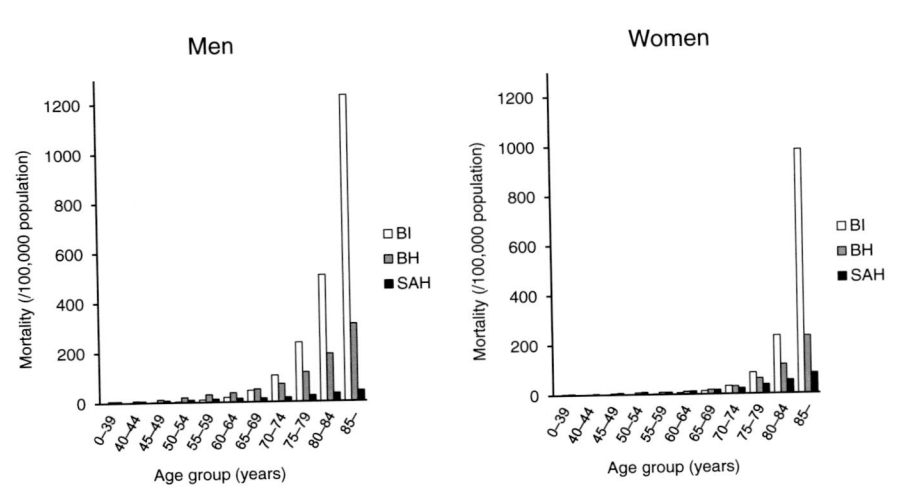

Fig. 9.2 Mortality of stroke in Japan according to age. Deaths (per 100,000 population) caused by brain infarction (BI, white bars), brain hemorrhage (BH, shaded bars), and subarachnoid hemorrhage (SAH, black bars), shown according to each age group for men and women (Vital Statistics 2010, Ministry of Health, Labour and Welfare)

9.2 Stroke Risk Factors and Prevention in the Elderly Population

9.2.1 Hypertension

High blood pressure is the most influential risk factor for the development of stroke. Prospective cohort studies have shown that the association between high blood pressure and stroke risk is present in all ages, even in people aged ≥80 years [11]. However, the cutoff value of systolic hypertension in relation to mortality may differ by age [12]. The increase in stroke risk per blood pressure change is less remarkable in old age than in middle age [11].

9.2.1.1 Antihypertensive Treatment

The question arises as to whether antihypertensive treatment can reduce stroke risk or mortality, even in elderly patients. In a meta-analysis of nine randomized controlled trials of antihypertensive treatment among patients aged ≥60 years, antihypertensive treatment reduced stroke morbidity and mortality by 35% and 36%, respectively [13]. In a meta-analysis of eight trials among patients aged ≥60 years who had isolated systolic hypertension ≥160 mmHg and diastolic blood pressure <95 mmHg, active treatment reduced total mortality by 13% and stroke by 30%; the absolute benefit was larger in patients aged ≥70 years [14]. To elucidate the benefits and risks of antihypertensive treatment in very old patients, the Hypertension in the Very Elderly Trial (HYVET) was performed among patients aged ≥80 years with sustained systolic blood pressure ≥160 mmHg. Consequently, active treatment with indapamide (and perindopril if necessary), targeting blood pressure of 150/80 mmHg, reduced the rate of fatal or nonfatal stroke and death from stroke by 30% and 39%, respectively [15]. Therefore, antihypertensive treatment seems to be beneficial, even in older patients.

9.2.1.2 Target Blood Pressure Levels

The optimal blood pressure level to reduce cardiovascular events without increasing adverse events remains uncertain in elderly patients. The presence of a J-shaped curve relationship between blood pressure and cardiovascular events remains a subject of debate [16]. Post hoc analysis of the Perindopril Protection Against Recurrent Stroke Study (PROGRESS) among patients with cerebrovascular disease reported that intensive blood pressure lowering, even below 120 mmHg, produced a greater reduction of stroke risk [17]. In contrast, a post hoc observational analysis of the Prevention Regimen for Effectively Avoiding Second Strokes (PROFESS) trial for patients with recent noncardioembolic ischemic stroke revealed a J-shaped relationship between systolic blood pressure levels and recurrent stroke [18].

In the Action to Control Cardiovascular Risk in Diabetes (ACCORD) study [19] and the Systolic Blood Pressure Intervention Trial (SPRINT) [20], the rates of cardiovascular events were lower, but those of serious adverse events were higher under intensive therapy (systolic blood pressure <120 mmHg) than under standard therapy (<140 mmHg) for participants with high cardiovascular risk. Currently, the optimal level of blood pressure should be determined after individualized assessment in aged patients [21].

9.2.2 Diabetes Mellitus

Diabetes mellitus is another well-known risk factor for stroke, the prevalence of which increases with advancing age. In patients with diabetes, adjusted hazard ratios increased to 2.27 (95% CI 1.95–2.65) for ischemic stroke and 1.56 (95% CI 1.19–2.05) for hemorrhagic stroke in a meta-analysis by the Emerging Risk Factors Collaboration [22]. In the Hisayama study, the risk of ischemic stroke increased with both fasting (7.0 mmol/L) and 2-h postload (11.1 mmol/L) glucose levels [23]. As the prevalence of diabetes is increasing in all countries [24], preventive measures against diabetes are needed to reduce the global stroke burden.

9.2.2.1 Glycemic Control

Recent trials failed to provide evidence that intensive glycemic control reduces stroke risk in diabetic patients. In the UK Prospective Diabetes Study (UKPDS) 33, intensive glucose control did not decrease the risk of cardiovascular diseases in patients with type 2 diabetes [25]. Thereafter, randomized clinical trials, such as the Action in Diabetes and Vascular Disease, Preterax and Diamicron Modified Release Controlled Evaluation (ADVANCE) [26], Action to Control Cardiovascular Risk in Diabetes (ACCORD) [27], and Veterans Affairs Diabetes Trial (VADT) [28], have been performed to determine whether further intensive glucose control can reduce cardiovascular events. However, intensive control could not significantly reduce major cardiovascular events, including stroke. In meta-analyses of 5 randomized controlled trials [29] and 13 additional trials [30], intensive treatment was not associated with a reduction in the risk of nonfatal stroke or all strokes.

Appropriate glycemic control is essential to avoid microvascular diabetic complications or acute diabetic complications, such as dehydration, poor wound healing, and hyperglycemic hyperosmolar coma. However, intensive glycemic control may not necessarily result in a reduction of stroke risk in diabetic patients. Because elderly patients are at higher risk of hypoglycemia, glycemic goals might be relaxed for these patients [31, 32].

9.2.2.2 Multifactorial Intervention

To prevent stroke during remaining life expectancy, control of concomitant cardio-vascular risk factors by use of antihypertensive, lipid-lowering, and antithrombotic treatments is important for older patients with diabetes. In older adults, these risk factors are treated in consideration of the life expectancy of each individual patient. In older adults with diabetes, targets and therapeutic approaches should be chosen after assessment of coexisting chronic illnesses as well as cognitive and functional status [31, 32].

9.2.3 Atrial Fibrillation

Atrial fibrillation could generate thrombus in the left atrium or appendage, which occasionally causes cardioembolic stroke. The incidence of atrial fibrillation increases with advancing age [33]; for instance, the age-specific prevalence in people aged 60–69, 70–79, and ≥80 years in Japan has been reported as 1.9, 3.4, and 4.4 in men and 0.4, 1.1, and 2.2 in women, respectively [34]. Additionally, stroke events significantly increase in older patients with atrial fibrillation. The Framingham study revealed that the attributable risk of stroke for atrial fibrillation was 1.5%, 2.8%, 9.9%, and 23.5% in people aged 50–59, 60–69, 70–79, and 80–89 years, respectively [35].

Risk stratification for stroke or systemic embolisms in patients with nonvalvular atrial fibrillation has been attempted, and risk scores have been developed. Among these, the $CHADS_2$ score (0–6 points) assigns 1 point for ages ≥75 years [36], and the CHA_2DS_2-VASc score (0–9 points) assigns 1 point for ages 64–74 years and 2 points for ages ≥75 years [37]. As underdiagnosis of atrial fibrillation appears to be a predominant cause of cardioembolic stroke [38], awareness, pulse palpitation, or electrocardiogram may be more necessary for the detection of atrial fibrillation in older populations.

9.2.3.1 Anticoagulation Therapy

Anticoagulation therapy is highly effective to reduce the risk of stroke in patients with atrial fibrillation. In people with atrial fibrillation aged >75 years, the event rate per 100 person-years is 3.22 in patients not taking warfarin but 1.43 in those taking warfarin [39]. Meta-analysis of 29 trials showed that adjusted-dose warfarin reduced stroke by 64% compared with controls [40]. As a result, according to the Framingham Heart study [41], the risk of stroke in the 20 years after onset of atrial fibrillation was reduced by 74% between 1958–1967 and 1998–2007.

Direct oral anticoagulants (DOACs; dabigatran [42], rivaroxaban [43], apixaban [44], edoxaban [45]) have been developed as alternatives for vitamin K antagonists in the prevention of stroke or systemic embolism in patients with atrial fibrillation. Subanalyses of trials investigating the risks of ischemic stroke and intracranial bleeding during treatment with DOACs in older patients have been conducted. In the Randomized Evaluation of Long-Term Anticoagulation Therapy (RE-LY) study, intracranial bleeding risk was lower, but extracranial bleeding risk was similar or higher in patients aged ≥75 years treated with dabigatran compared with those taking warfarin [46]. In the trial entitled Rivaroxaban Once Daily Oral Direct Factor Xa Inhibition Compared with Vitamin K Antagonism for Prevention of Stroke and Embolism Trial in Atrial Fibrillation (ROCKET AF), the risk of major bleeding increased with age, but there were no apparent differences in the risk of major bleeding between rivaroxaban and warfarin in each age category (<65, 65–74, ≥75 years) [47]. In the Apixaban for Reduction in Stroke and Other Thromboembolic Events in Atrial Fibrillation (ARISTOTLE) trial, the rates of stroke or systemic embolism and major bleeding were lower in the apixaban group than in the warfarin group, regardless of age [44, 48]. The net clinical benefit for older patients should be compared between DOACs and vitamin K antagonists in the real-world setting.

9.2.3.2 Hemorrhagic Risk During Anticoagulation Therapy

Old age is an important risk factor for major bleeding during anticoagulation therapy. Age (years of age, ABC score [49]; age >65 years, HAS-BLED score [50]; age ≥75 years, HEMORR$_2$HAGES score [51], ATRIA score [52], and ORBIT score [53]) is included as an item in the risk scores for bleeding during anticoagulation.

The incidence of hemorrhagic stroke has been reported as high in Asian people [3]. The reported incidence of intracerebral hemorrhage per 100,000 person-years is 24.2 (95% CI 20.9–28.0) in white people, 22.9 (95% CI 14.8–35.6) in blacks, 19.6 (95% CI 15.7–24.5) in Hispanic populations, and 51.8 (95% CI 38.8–69.3) in Asians [54]. Similarly, the hazard ratio of intracranial hemorrhage during warfarin therapy for atrial fibrillation increased to 4.06 (95% CI 2.47–6.65) in Asians compared with whites as referent [55]. Previous studies in Japanese patients with atrial fibrillation revealed that the optimal prothrombin time (PT)-international normalized ratio (INR) to reduce the risk of major ischemic or hemorrhagic events may be lower in older patients than in younger ones [56, 57]. Based on these findings, Japanese guidelines for pharmacotherapy for atrial fibrillation recommend warfarin therapy with a target PT-INR range of 1.6–2.6 for patients aged ≥70 years and a target of 2.0–3.0 for patients aged <70 years [58]. In older patients, careful monitoring of the intensity of anticoagulation is crucial to extend the time maintained in the therapeutic range to as long as possible.

9.2.4 Hypercholesterolemia

Hypercholesterolemia is known as a risk factor for major coronary events; however, the association between cholesterol levels and stroke is inconsistent or weak. The association may be evident if we investigate the relationship of LDL cholesterol levels with ischemic stroke caused by thrombotic mechanisms. In the Hisayama study, the age- and sex-adjusted incidences were significantly elevated for athero-thrombotic and lacunar infarctions with increasing LDL cholesterol level [59].

9.2.4.1   Lipid-Lowering Treatment

Lipid-lowering treatment with statins is considered effective in reducing both initial and recurrent stroke. The Stroke Prevention by Aggressive Reduction in Cholesterol Levels (SPARCL) trial revealed that 80 mg of atorvastatin reduced the overall incidence of stroke in patients with a recent stroke or TIA [60]. Meta-analysis of randomized trials of statins showed that each 1-mmol/L decrease in LDL cholesterol equates to a reduction in relative risk for stroke of 21.1% (95% CI 6.3–33.5). In secondary prevention of noncardioembolic stroke, intense reduction of LDL cholesterol by statins also reduced the risk of recurrent stroke (relative risk [RR] 0.84, 95% CI 0.71–0.99) [61].

A meta-analysis of individual data from 61 prospective studies suggested that total cholesterol was negatively related to hemorrhagic and total stroke mortality, particularly in patients with older ages (70–89 years) and systolic blood pressure >145 mmHg [62]. However, other meta-analyses of randomized trials did not show a significant increase in the risk of hemorrhagic stroke by intense lipid lowering [61, 63]. Recently, the Improved Reduction of Outcomes: Vytorin Efficacy International Trial (IMPROVE-IT) demonstrated that the risk of cardiovascular events was further lowered by the addition of ezetimibe to simvastatin therapy, with a nonsignificantly high risk of hemorrhagic stroke in stable patients with an acute coronary syndrome [64]. In elderly patients without established cardiovascular disease, statins reduced the incidence of myocardial infarction and stroke, but did not significantly prolong their survival in the short term.[65] Further studies are still needed to clarify the benefit of lipid-lowering therapy in older people, especially those without diabetes or cardiovascular risk factors.

9.3   Stroke Treatment for Elderly Patients

9.3.1   Stroke Care Unit

Poststroke functional outcome becomes worse with increasing age. We previously showed that women had higher risk of poor outcome after stroke than men, among patients aged ≥70 years [66]. To improve poststroke functional outcome in elderly patients, stroke care units may be beneficial. Randomized trials have been conducted on the efficacy of stroke units, and meta-analysis revealed that organized stroke unit care results in reductions in death, dependency, and the need for institutional care [67, 68]. In older patients aged ≥70 years with acute stroke and concomitant cardiac disease, the risk of death or institutional care was reduced after 3 months among patients in the stroke unit compared with those receiving conventional care [69]. A quasi-randomized, controlled study among patients ≥60 years old with stroke within 24 h of onset revealed that treatment in the stroke unit increased survival at 12 and 18 months after stroke onset and patients with intracerebral hemorrhage benefitted the most [70]. Benefits of the stroke unit likely exist for elderly patients, but the effects on clinically reliable outcomes are modest and insignificant [71].

9.3.2 Intravenous Thrombolytic Therapy

Intravenous recombinant tissue plasminogen activator (rt-PA) is highly effective in improving functional outcome after acute ischemic stroke. However, there are a number of clinical, radiological, and laboratory-related exclusion criteria for rt-PA because of the potential risk of hemorrhagic events [72]. In a post hoc subgroup analysis of the National Institute of Neurological Disorders and Stroke (NINDS) t-PA stroke trial for stroke patients within 3 h of symptom onset, there was no favorable response to treatment in patients aged >75 years [73]. Therefore, advanced age is recognized as a factor related to increased hemorrhagic risk with little benefit of rt-PA.

However, recent analysis of the Safe Implementation of Treatments in Stroke, a prospective internet-based audit of the International Stroke Thrombolysis Registry (SITS-ISTR) and the Virtual International Stroke Trials Archive (VISTA), demonstrated that the association between thrombolysis treatment and improved outcome was maintained in very elderly people [74]. Furthermore, the third International Stroke Trial (IST-3) indicated greater benefit in patients >80 years of age, contrary to expectations [75]. Systematic review and meta-analysis showed that the effect of rt-PA treatment was similar between patients aged ≤80 years and those >80 years [76, 77]. We also investigated the efficacy and safety of intravenous rt-PA in elderly Japanese patients by propensity score (PS)-matched case-control analysis. Consequently, intravenous rt-PA therapy was associated with improved clinical outcomes without a significant increase in risk of hemorrhagic complications in elderly patients aged >80 years with acute ischemic stroke [78]. Thus, age alone may not be a contraindication to the treatment. Nevertheless, use of intravenous rt-PA should be cautiously considered after estimating the balance between benefits and risks of therapy for elderly patients.

9.3.3 Carotid Endarterectomy and Stenting

Carotid endarterectomy (CEA) and endovascular carotid artery stenting (CAS) reduce the risk of ischemic stroke in patients with carotid stenosis. However, the benefit and safety of these procedures may differ depending on the patient's age. In the North American Symptomatic Carotid Endarterectomy Trial (NASCET), the risk of ipsilateral ischemic stroke at 2 years was decreased by CEA in three age categories (<65, 65–74, and ≥75 years) for patients with 70–99% stenosis [79]. Further analysis of pooled data from the European Carotid Surgery Trial (ECST) and NASCET showed that the benefit from surgery was greatest in patients aged ≥75 years [80]. Moreover, in patients with 50–69% stenosis, the absolute risk reduction was significant only in those aged ≥75 years [79].

Many studies have been done to compare the benefit and safety of CEA and CAS in elderly patients. In post hoc analyses of data in the Stent-Protected Angioplasty versus Carotid Endarterectomy in Symptomatic Patients (SPACE) trial, the risk of ipsilateral stroke or death significantly increased with age in the CAS group but not in the CEA group [81]. The pooled data from the Endarterectomy Versus Angioplasty in Patients with Symptomatic Severe Carotid Stenosis (EVA-3S), SPACE, and the International Carotid Stenting Study (ICSS) favored CEA more strongly with increasing age, although risk ratios of any stroke or death within 120 days of randomization increased linearly with age [82]. CAS tended to show greater efficacy at younger ages, and CEA at older ages, with a crossover at age approximately 70 years [83]. In the Carotid Revascularization Endarterectomy versus Stenting Trial (CREST), risk for the primary end point, including stroke, increased with age by 1.77 (95% CI 1.38–2.28) per 10-year increment for CAS, whereas there was no evidence of increased risk for CEA-treated patients [84]. In the meta-analysis of individual patient-level data from the Carotid Stenosis Trialists' Collaboration (CSTC), the periprocedural risk for stroke and death in patients receiving CAS was roughly 4.0 for age ≥70 years compared with age <60 years, although there was no evidence of an increased periprocedural risk by age group in the CEA group [85].

Recently, embolic protection devices have been developed, which reduce the stroke risk during the procedure. Moreover, the best medical treatment in recent years is more effective than before to decrease stroke risk, possibly via stabilization and regression of plaque with carotid stenosis. Carotid stenosis should be treated based on up-to-date evidence in elderly patients.

9.4   Conclusions

A number of studies have revealed the benefits and risks of stroke prevention and stroke care in the elderly population. To effectively prevent stroke and improve poststroke outcomes in older patients, appropriate health care should be provided that is based on the latest evidence, in consideration of each person's age, disability, frailty, comorbidity, and cardiovascular risk.

Acknowledgments   This work was supported by the Japan Society for the Promotion of Science (JSPS) KAKENHI grant number 17H04143.

References

1. Hata J, Ninomiya T, Hirakawa Y, Nagata M, Mukai N, Gotoh S, et al. Secular trends in cardiovascular disease and its risk factors in Japanese: half-century data from the Hisayama study (1961–2009). Circulation. 2013;128(11):1198–205.
2. Kubo M, Kiyohara Y, Kato I, Tanizaki Y, Arima H, Tanaka K, et al. Trends in the incidence, mortality, and survival rate of cardiovascular disease in a Japanese community: the Hisayama study. Stroke. 2003;34(10):2349–54.
3. Krishnamurthi RV, Feigin VL, Forouzanfar MH, Mensah GA, Connor M, Bennett DA, et al. Global and regional burden of first-ever ischaemic and haemorrhagic stroke during 1990–2010: findings from the Global Burden of Disease Study 2010. Lancet Glob Health. 2013;1(5):e259–81.
4. Kamouchi M, Kumagai N, Okada Y, Origasa H, Yamaguchi T, Kitazono T. Risk score for predicting recurrence in patients with ischemic stroke: the Fukuoka stroke risk score for Japanese. Cerebrovasc Dis. 2012;34(5–6):351–7.
5. Rothwell PM, Giles MF, Flossmann E, Lovelock CE, Redgrave JN, Warlow CP, et al. A simple score (ABCD) to identify individuals at high early risk of stroke after transient ischaemic attack. Lancet. 2005;366(9479):29–36.
6. Johnston SC, Rothwell PM, Nguyen-Huynh MN, Giles MF, Elkins JS, Bernstein AL, et al. Validation and refinement of scores to predict very early stroke risk after transient ischaemic attack. Lancet. 2007;369(9558):283–92.
7. Kiyohara T, Kamouchi M, Kumai Y, Ninomiya T, Hata J, Yoshimura S, et al. ABCD3 and ABCD3-I scores are superior to ABCD2 score in the prediction of short- and long-term risks of stroke after transient ischemic attack. Stroke. 2014;45(2):418–25.
8. Feigin VL, Forouzanfar MH, Krishnamurthi R, Mensah GA, Connor M, Bennett DA, et al. Global and regional burden of stroke during 1990–2010: findings from the Global Burden of Disease Study 2010. Lancet. 2014;383(9913):245–54.
9. Fonarow GC, Reeves MJ, Zhao X, Olson DM, Smith EE, Saver JL, et al. Age-related differences in characteristics, performance measures, treatment trends, and outcomes in patients with ischemic stroke. Circulation. 2010;121(7):879–91.
10. Lackland DT, Roccella EJ, Deutsch AF, Fornage M, George MG, Howard G, et al. Factors influencing the decline in stroke mortality: a statement from the American Heart Association/American Stroke Association. Stroke. 2014;45(1):315–53.
11. Lawes CM, Bennett DA, Feigin VL, Rodgers A. Blood pressure and stroke: an overview of published reviews. Stroke. 2004;35(4):1024.
12. Port S, Demer L, Jennrich R, Walter D, Garfinkel A. Systolic blood pressure and mortality. Lancet. 2000;355(9199):175–80.
13. Insua JT, Sacks HS, Lau TS, Lau J, Reitman D, Pagano D, et al. Drug treatment of hypertension in the elderly: a meta-analysis. Ann Intern Med. 1994;121(5):355–62.
14. Staessen JA, Gasowski J, Wang JG, Thijs L, Den Hond E, Boissel JP, et al. Risks of untreated and treated isolated systolic hypertension in the elderly: meta-analysis of outcome trials. Lancet. 2000;355(9207):865–72.
15. Beckett NS, Peters R, Fletcher AE, Staessen JA, Liu L, Dumitrascu D, et al. Treatment of hypertension in patients 80 years of age or older. N Engl J Med. 2008;358(18):1887–98.
16. Malyszko J, Muntner P, Rysz J, Banach M. Blood pressure levels and stroke: J-curve phenomenon? Curr Hypertens Rep. 2013;15(6):575–81.
17. Arima H, Chalmers J, Woodward M, Anderson C, Rodgers A, Davis S, et al. Lower target blood pressures are safe and effective for the prevention of recurrent stroke: the PROGRESS trial. J Hypertens. 2006;24(6):1201–8.
18. Ovbiagele B, Diener HC, Yusuf S, Martin RH, Cotton D, Vinisko R, et al. Level of systolic blood pressure within the normal range and risk of recurrent stroke. JAMA. 2011;306(19):2137–44.

19. Cushman WC, Evans GW, Byington RP, Goff DC Jr, Grimm RH Jr, Cutler JA, et al. Effects of intensive blood-pressure control in type 2 diabetes mellitus. N Engl J Med. 2010;362(17):1575–85.
20. Wright JT Jr, Williamson JD, Whelton PK, Snyder JK, Sink KM, Rocco MV, et al. A randomized trial of intensive versus standard blood-pressure control. N Engl J Med. 2015;373(22):2103–16.
21. Qaseem A, Wilt TJ, Rich R, Humphrey LL, Frost J, Forciea MA, et al. Pharmacologic treatment of hypertension in adults aged 60 years or older to higher versus lower blood pressure targets: a clinical practice guideline from the American College of Physicians and the American Academy of Family Physicians. Ann Intern Med. 2017;166(6):430–7.
22. Sarwar N, Gao P, Seshasai SR, Gobin R, Kaptoge S, Di Angelantonio E, et al. Diabetes mellitus, fasting blood glucose concentration, and risk of vascular disease: a collaborative meta-analysis of 102 prospective studies. Lancet. 2010;375(9733):2215–22.
23. Doi Y, Ninomiya T, Hata J, Fukuhara M, Yonemoto K, Iwase M, et al. Impact of glucose tolerance status on development of ischemic stroke and coronary heart disease in a general Japanese population: the Hisayama study. Stroke. 2010;41(2):203–9.
24. NCD Risk Factor Collaboration. Worldwide trends in diabetes since 1980: a pooled analysis of 751 population-based studies with 4.4 million participants. Lancet. 2016;387(10027):1513–30.
25. UK Prospective Diabetes Study (UKPDS) Group. Intensive blood-glucose control with sulphonylureas or insulin compared with conventional treatment and risk of complications in patients with type 2 diabetes (UKPDS 33). Lancet. 1998;352(9131):837–53.
26. Patel A, MacMahon S, Chalmers J, Neal B, Billot L, Woodward M, et al. Intensive blood glucose control and vascular outcomes in patients with type 2 diabetes. N Engl J Med. 2008;358(24):2560–72.
27. Gerstein HC, Miller ME, Byington RP, Goff DC Jr, Bigger JT, Buse JB, et al. Effects of intensive glucose lowering in type 2 diabetes. N Engl J Med. 2008;358(24):2545–59.
28. Duckworth W, Abraira C, Moritz T, Reda D, Emanuele N, Reaven PD, et al. Glucose control and vascular complications in veterans with type 2 diabetes. N Engl J Med. 2009;360(2):129–39.
29. Ray KK, Seshasai SR, Wijesuriya S, Sivakumaran R, Nethercott S, Preiss D, et al. Effect of intensive control of glucose on cardiovascular outcomes and death in patients with diabetes mellitus: a meta-analysis of randomised controlled trials. Lancet. 2009;373(9677):1765–72.
30. Boussageon R, Bejan-Angoulvant T, Saadatian-Elahi M, Lafont S, Bergeonneau C, Kassai B, et al. Effect of intensive glucose lowering treatment on all cause mortality, cardiovascular death, and microvascular events in type 2 diabetes: meta-analysis of randomised controlled trials. BMJ. 2011;343:d4169.
31. Kirkman MS, Briscoe VJ, Clark N, Florez H, Haas LB, Halter JB, et al. Diabetes in older adults. Diabetes Care. 2012;35(12):2650–64.
32. American Diabetes Association. 10. Older adults. Diabetes Care. 2016;39(Suppl 1):S81–5.
33. Rodriguez CJ, Soliman EZ, Alonso A, Swett K, Okin PM, Goff DC Jr, et al. Atrial fibrillation incidence and risk factors in relation to race-ethnicity and the population attributable fraction of atrial fibrillation risk factors: the Multi-Ethnic Study of Atherosclerosis. Ann Epidemiol. 2015;25(2):71–6, 6.e1.
34. Inoue H, Fujiki A, Origasa H, Ogawa S, Okumura K, Kubota I, et al. Prevalence of atrial fibrillation in the general population of Japan: an analysis based on periodic health examination. Int J Cardiol. 2009;137(2):102–7.
35. Wolf PA, Abbott RD, Kannel WB. Atrial fibrillation as an independent risk factor for stroke: the Framingham study. Stroke. 1991;22(8):983–8.
36. Gage BF, Waterman AD, Shannon W, Boechler M, Rich MW, Radford MJ. Validation of clinical classification schemes for predicting stroke: results from the National Registry of Atrial Fibrillation. JAMA. 2001;285(22):2864–70.
37. Lip GY, Nieuwlaat R, Pisters R, Lane DA, Crijns HJ. Refining clinical risk stratification for predicting stroke and thromboembolism in atrial fibrillation using a novel risk factor-based approach: the Euro Heart Survey on atrial fibrillation. Chest. 2010;137(2):263–72.

38. Nakamura A, Kuroda J, Ago T, Hata J, Matsuo R, Arakawa S, et al. Causes of ischemic stroke in patients with non-valvular atrial fibrillation. Cerebrovasc Dis. 2016;42(3–4):196–204.

39. Go AS, Hylek EM, Chang Y, Phillips KA, Henault LE, Capra AM, et al. Anticoagulation therapy for stroke prevention in atrial fibrillation: how well do randomized trials translate into clinical practice? JAMA. 2003;290(20):2685–92.

40. Hart RG, Pearce LA, Aguilar MI. Meta-analysis: antithrombotic therapy to prevent stroke in patients who have nonvalvular atrial fibrillation. Ann Intern Med. 2007;146(12):857–67.

41. Schnabel RB, Yin X, Gona P, Larson MG, Beiser AS, McManus DD, et al. 50 Year trends in atrial fibrillation prevalence, incidence, risk factors, and mortality in the Framingham Heart Study: a cohort study. Lancet. 2015;386(9989):154–62.

42. Connolly SJ, Ezekowitz MD, Yusuf S, Eikelboom J, Oldgren J, Parekh A, et al. Dabigatran versus warfarin in patients with atrial fibrillation. N Engl J Med. 2009;361(12):1139–51.

43. Patel MR, Mahaffey KW, Garg J, Pan G, Singer DE, Hacke W, et al. Rivaroxaban versus warfarin in nonvalvular atrial fibrillation. N Engl J Med. 2011;365(10):883–91.

44. Granger CB, Alexander JH, McMurray JJ, Lopes RD, Hylek EM, Hanna M, et al. Apixaban versus warfarin in patients with atrial fibrillation. N Engl J Med. 2011;365(11):981–92.

45. Giugliano RP, Ruff CT, Braunwald E, Murphy SA, Wiviott SD, Halperin JL, et al. Edoxaban versus warfarin in patients with atrial fibrillation. N Engl J Med. 2013;369(22):2093–104.

46. Eikelboom JW, Wallentin L, Connolly SJ, Ezekowitz M, Healey JS, Oldgren J, et al. Risk of bleeding with 2 doses of dabigatran compared with warfarin in older and younger patients with atrial fibrillation: an analysis of the randomized evaluation of long-term anticoagulant therapy (RE-LY) trial. Circulation. 2011;123(21):2363–72.

47. Goodman SG, Wojdyla DM, Piccini JP, White HD, Paolini JF, Nessel CC, et al. Factors associated with major bleeding events: insights from the ROCKET AF trial (rivaroxaban once-daily oral direct factor Xa inhibition compared with vitamin K antagonism for prevention of stroke and embolism trial in atrial fibrillation). J Am Coll Cardiol. 2014;63(9):891–900.

48. Halvorsen S, Atar D, Yang H, De Caterina R, Erol C, Garcia D, et al. Efficacy and safety of apixaban compared with warfarin according to age for stroke prevention in atrial fibrillation: observations from the ARISTOTLE trial. Eur Heart J. 2014;35(28):1864–72.

49. Hijazi Z, Oldgren J, Lindback J, Alexander JH, Connolly SJ, Eikelboom JW, et al. The novel biomarker-based ABC (age, biomarkers, clinical history)-bleeding risk score for patients with atrial fibrillation: a derivation and validation study. Lancet. 2016;387(10035):2302–11.

50. Pisters R, Lane DA, Nieuwlaat R, de Vos CB, Crijns HJ, Lip GY. A novel user-friendly score (HAS-BLED) to assess 1-year risk of major bleeding in patients with atrial fibrillation: the Euro Heart Survey. Chest. 2010;138(5):1093–100.

51. Gage BF, Yan Y, Milligan PE, Waterman AD, Culverhouse R, Rich MW, et al. Clinical classification schemes for predicting hemorrhage: results from the National Registry of Atrial Fibrillation (NRAF). Am Heart J. 2006;151(3):713–9.

52. Fang MC, Go AS, Chang Y, Borowsky LH, Pomernacki NK, Udaltsova N, et al. A new risk scheme to predict warfarin-associated hemorrhage: the ATRIA (anticoagulation and risk factors in atrial fibrillation) study. J Am Coll Cardiol. 2011;58(4):395–401.

53. O'Brien EC, Simon DN, Thomas LE, Hylek EM, Gersh BJ, Ansell JE, et al. The ORBIT bleeding score: a simple bedside score to assess bleeding risk in atrial fibrillation. Eur Heart J. 2015;36(46):3258–64.

54. van Asch CJ, Luitse MJ, Rinkel GJ, van der Tweel I, Algra A, Klijn CJ. Incidence, case fatality, and functional outcome of intracerebral haemorrhage over time, according to age, sex, and ethnic origin: a systematic review and meta-analysis. Lancet Neurol. 2010;9(2):167–76.

55. Shen AY, Yao JF, Brar SS, Jorgensen MB, Chen W. Racial/ethnic differences in the risk of intracranial hemorrhage among patients with atrial fibrillation. J Am Coll Cardiol. 2007;50(4):309–15.

56. Yasaka M, Minematsu K, Yamaguchi T. Optimal intensity of international normalized ratio in warfarin therapy for secondary prevention of stroke in patients with non-valvular atrial fibrillation. Intern Med. 2001;40(12):1183–8.

57. Yamaguchi T. Optimal intensity of warfarin therapy for secondary prevention of stroke in patients with nonvalvular atrial fibrillation: a multicenter, prospective, randomized trial. Japanese Nonvalvular Atrial Fibrillation-Embolism Secondary Prevention Cooperative Study Group. Stroke. 2000;31(4):817–21.
58. JCS Joint Working Group. Guidelines for pharmacotherapy of atrial fibrillation (JCS 2013). Circ J. 2014;78(8):1997–2021.
59. Imamura T, Doi Y, Arima H, Yonemoto K, Hata J, Kubo M, et al. LDL cholesterol and the development of stroke subtypes and coronary heart disease in a general Japanese population: the Hisayama study. Stroke. 2009;40(2):382–8.
60. Amarenco P, Bogousslavsky J, Callahan A 3rd, Goldstein LB, Hennerici M, Rudolph AE, et al. High-dose atorvastatin after stroke or transient ischemic attack. N Engl J Med. 2006;355(6):549–59.
61. Amarenco P, Labreuche J. Lipid management in the prevention of stroke: review and updated meta-analysis of statins for stroke prevention. Lancet Neurol. 2009;8(5):453–63.
62. Lewington S, Whitlock G, Clarke R, Sherliker P, Emberson J, Halsey J, et al. Blood cholesterol and vascular mortality by age, sex, and blood pressure: a meta-analysis of individual data from 61 prospective studies with 55,000 vascular deaths. Lancet. 2007;370(9602):1829–39.
63. Baigent C, Blackwell L, Emberson J, Holland LE, Reith C, Bhala N, et al. Efficacy and safety of more intensive lowering of LDL cholesterol: a meta-analysis of data from 170,000 participants in 26 randomised trials. Lancet. 2010;376(9753):1670–81.
64. Cannon CP, Blazing MA, Giugliano RP, McCagg A, White JA, Theroux P, et al. Ezetimibe added to statin therapy after acute coronary syndromes. N Engl J Med. 2015;372(25):2387–97.
65. Savarese G, Gotto AM Jr, Paolillo S, D'Amore C, Losco T, Musella F, et al. Benefits of statins in elderly subjects without established cardiovascular disease: a meta-analysis. J Am Coll Cardiol. 2013;62(22):2090–9.
66. Irie F, Kamouchi M, Hata J, Matsuo R, Wakisaka Y, Kuroda J, et al. Sex differences in short-term outcomes after acute ischemic stroke: the Fukuoka Stroke Registry. Stroke. 2015;46(2):471–6.
67. Stroke Unit Trialists Collaboration. How do stroke units improve patient outcomes? A collaborative systematic review of the randomized trials. Stroke. 1997;28(11):2139–44.
68. Stroke Unit Trialists' Collaboration. Collaborative systematic review of the randomised trials of organised inpatient (stroke unit) care after stroke. BMJ. 1997;314(7088):1151–9.
69. Fagerberg B, Claesson L, Gosman-Hedström G, Blomstrand C. Effect of acute stroke unit care integrated with care continuum versus conventional treatment: a randomized 1-year study of elderly patients: the Göteborg 70+ stroke study. Stroke. 2000;31(11):2578–84.
70. Rønning OM, Guldvog B. Stroke units versus general medical wards, I: twelve- and eighteen-month survival: a randomized, controlled trial. Stroke. 1998;29(1):58–62.
71. Rønning OM, Guldvog B. Stroke unit versus general medical wards, II: neurological deficits and activities of daily living: a quasi-randomized controlled trial. Stroke. 1998;29(3):586–90.
72. Demaerschalk BM, Kleindorfer DO, Adeoye OM, Demchuk AM, Fugate JE, Grotta JC, et al. Scientific rationale for the inclusion and exclusion criteria for intravenous alteplase in acute ischemic stroke: a statement for healthcare professionals from the American Heart Association/American Stroke Association. Stroke. 2016;47(2):581–641.
73. The NINDS t-PA Stroke Study Group. Generalized efficacy of t-PA for acute stroke. Subgroup analysis of the NINDS t-PA Stroke Trial. Stroke. 1997;28(11):2119–25.
74. Mishra NK, Ahmed N, Andersen G, Egido JA, Lindsberg PJ, Ringleb PA, et al. Thrombolysis in very elderly people: controlled comparison of SITS International Stroke Thrombolysis Registry and Virtual International Stroke Trials Archive. BMJ. 2010;341:c6046.
75. Sandercock P, Wardlaw JM, Lindley RI, Dennis M, Cohen G, Murray G, et al. The benefits and harms of intravenous thrombolysis with recombinant tissue plasminogen activator within 6 h of acute ischaemic stroke (the third international stroke trial [IST-3]): a randomised controlled trial. Lancet. 2012;379(9834):2352–63.

76. Wardlaw JM, Murray V, Berge E, del Zoppo G, Sandercock P, Lindley RL, et al. Recombinant tissue plasminogen activator for acute ischaemic stroke: an updated systematic review and meta-analysis. Lancet. 2012;379(9834):2364–72.
77. Emberson J, Lees KR, Lyden P, Blackwell L, Albers G, Bluhmki E, et al. Effect of treatment delay, age, and stroke severity on the effects of intravenous thrombolysis with alteplase for acute ischaemic stroke: a meta-analysis of individual patient data from randomised trials. Lancet. 2014;384(9958):1929–35.
78. Matsuo R, Kamouchi M, Fukuda H, Hata J, Wakisaka Y, Kuroda J, et al. Intravenous thrombolysis with recombinant tissue plasminogen activator for ischemic stroke patients over 80 years old: the Fukuoka Stroke Registry. PLoS One. 2014;9(10):e110444.
79. Alamowitch S, Eliasziw M, Algra A, Meldrum H, Barnett HJ. North American Symptomatic Carotid Endarterectomy Trial Group. Risk, causes, and prevention of ischaemic stroke in elderly patients with symptomatic internal-carotid-artery stenosis. Lancet. 2001;357(9263):1154–60.
80. Rothwell PM, Eliasziw M, Gutnikov SA, Warlow CP, Barnett HJ, Carotid Endarterectomy Trialists Collaboration. Endarterectomy for symptomatic carotid stenosis in relation to clinical subgroups and timing of surgery. Lancet. 2004;363(9413):915–24.
81. Stingele R, Berger J, Alfke K, Eckstein HH, Fraedrich G, Allenberg J, et al. Clinical and angiographic risk factors for stroke and death within 30 days after carotid endarterectomy and stent-protected angioplasty: a subanalysis of the SPACE study. Lancet Neurol. 2008;7(3):216–22.
82. Bonati LH, Dobson J, Algra A, Branchereau A, Chatellier G, Fraedrich G, et al. Short-term outcome after stenting versus endarterectomy for symptomatic carotid stenosis: a preplanned meta-analysis of individual patient data. Lancet. 2010;376(9746):1062–73.
83. Brott TG, Hobson RW 2nd, Howard G, Roubin GS, Clark WM, Brooks W, et al. Stenting versus endarterectomy for treatment of carotid-artery stenosis. N Engl J Med. 2010;363(1):11–23.
84. Voeks JH, Howard G, Roubin GS, Malas MB, Cohen DJ, Sternbergh WC 3rd, et al. Age and outcomes after carotid stenting and endarterectomy: the Carotid Revascularization Endarterectomy Versus Stenting Trial. Stroke. 2011;42(12):3484–90.
85. Howard G, Roubin GS, Jansen O, Hendrikse J, Halliday A, Fraedrich G, et al. Association between age and risk of stroke or death from carotid endarterectomy and carotid stenting: a meta-analysis of pooled patient data from four randomised trials. Lancet. 2016;387(10025):1305–11.

Chapter 10
Chronic Kidney Disease (CKD) as an Emerging Risk Factor in the Elderly

Kunitoshi Iseki

Abstract Chronic kidney disease (CKD) is becoming an increasingly prevalent clinical entity, and its severity is defined by the combination of albuminuria (proteinuria) and the glomerular filtration rate (GFR). Chronicity denotes 3 months and longer. CKD was first recognized as a risk factor for CVD by cardiologists, but the association of CKD with many other diseases, such as bone, muscle, and gastrointestinal diseases, stroke (cognitive function), malignancies, and infection, has become increasingly recognized.

The term "elderly" is used for persons ≥65 years of age, whereas "very elderly" is reserved for persons ≥80 years of age. Chronologic age is used as a surrogate for biologic age, although this relationship is highly variable. The leading cause of end-stage renal disease (ESRD) requiring dialysis therapy is DM, which accounts for approximately 44% of the total in Japan.

The elderly population is rapidly increasing in both developed and developing countries, and Japan has the highest rate of increase. The screening system for CKD is highly developed in Japan and begins with school children through the general population. Signs and symptoms associated with normal aging may, at least partly, be explained by the physiologic decline in the GFR.

The clinical relevance of CKD among the elderly population is becoming more evident. More studies of patient reported outcomes are needed for the development of clinical practice guidelines.

Keywords Proteinuria · Glomerular filtration rate (GFR) · Chronic kidney disease (CKD) · Cardiovascular disease (CVD) · End-stage renal disease (ESRD)

K. Iseki
Clinical Research Support Center, Nakamura Clinic, Okinawa, Japan

© Springer Nature Singapore Pte Ltd. 2019
M. Washio, C. Kiyohara (eds.), *Health Issues and Care System for the Elderly*,
Current Topics in Environmental Health and Preventive Medicine,
https://doi.org/10.1007/978-981-13-1762-0_10

10.1 Introduction

Chronic kidney disease (CKD) is becoming an increasingly prevalent clinical entity, and its severity is defined by the combination of albuminuria (proteinuria) and the glomerular filtration rate (GFR) [1]. Chronicity denotes 3 months and longer. As people age, the incidence of lifestyle-related disease such as hypertension, diabetes mellitus (DM), dyslipidemia, and hyperuricemia increases, and many die due to cardiovascular disease (CVD), infection, and malignancy. Kidney disease was first recognized as a risk factor for CVD by cardiologists [2], but the association of CKD with many other diseases, such as bone, muscle, and gastrointestinal diseases, stroke (cognitive function), malignancies, and infection, has become increasingly recognized.

Many patients with CKD have accumulated comorbidities associated with aging, including vascular disease, osteoporosis, and general frailty. The term "elderly" is used for persons ≥65 years of age, whereas "very elderly" is reserved for persons ≥80 years of age. Chronologic age is used as a surrogate for biologic age, although this relationship is highly variable of the Japanese Society for Dialysis Therapy (JSDT), the mean age at the start of dialysis therapy is increasing and is currently more than 68 years [3]. The leading cause of end-stage renal disease (ESRD) requiring dialysis therapy is DM, which accounts for approximately 44% of the total. In patients with nephrosclerosis, mean age at the start of dialysis is approximately 75 years. In 2015, the prevalence of dialysis among the very elderly (≥75 years old) was 29.4% in men and 36.6% in women.

10.2 Clinical Topics

10.2.1 Aging and CKD

The glomerular filtration rate (GFR) decreases with aging. Estimated GFR (eGFR), based on age, sex, and serum creatinine, is convenient for clinical use. The formula devised by the Japanese Society of Nephrology [4] is applied to Japanese patients and verified with a gold standard method such as inulin clearance. This formula may not be applicable for subjects who are malnourished, very elderly, or obese. The mechanisms of the physiologic decline in kidney function are not clear. The rate of eGFR decline is estimated to be approximately 8 mL/min/1.73 m^2 over 10 years. Therefore, the eGFR of aged people is expected to be approximately 60 mL/min/1.73 m^2 in someone whose eGFR was 100 mL/min/1.73 m^2 at 20 years of age. The number of nephrons does not increase after birth and depends on the birthweight. Maternal condition is partly defined by ethnic factors, genetics, and nutritional status. In contrast to Caucasian people, few studies of Asian populations are available.

We reported that the prevalence of CKD (eGFR <60 mL/min/1.73 m²) increases with age [5]. CKD is observed in more than 30% of both men and women 75 years age and over. The rate of decline of GFR is significantly higher in participants with an initial GFR <50 mL/min/1.73 m² among subjects younger than 70 years of age and in participants with an initial GFR <40 mL/min/1.73 m² in subjects 70–79 years of age. Based on the slow rate of GFR decline, we concluded that the decline in renal function progresses slowly in the Japanese general population [6]. Hypertension, proteinuria, and lower GFR are significant risk factors for a faster decline in GFR.

In advanced CKD (stage 3b–4), uremic symptoms appear, such as fatigue, anorexia, nausea, vomiting, and itching, but these symptoms are not specific to uremia, and some patients with CKD remain asymptomatic up to stage 5 CKD. Therefore, renal function should not only be assessed using only serum creatinine levels but should also be assessed using a predictive equation based on serum creatinine values [7]. The time to initiate hemodialysis should be determined by comprehensively assessing the serum creatinine levels, changes in GFR over time, and the physical constitution, age, sex, and nutritional condition of the patient, particularly in elderly patients.

10.2.2 Factors of CKD

Yamagata et al. examined the risk factors for developing CKD among general screened subjects in Ibaraki, Japan [8]. In addition to age, hypertension, DM, hypercholesterolemia, hypertriglyceridemia, obesity, and smoking [9], dipstick-positive proteinuria is a risk factor. A moderate intake of alcohol, less than 20 g/day, was rather protective against developing proteinuria. This favorable effect was diminished, however, by an alcohol intake of more than 20 g/day. The risk factors for reduced eGFR were similar, except for DM. In subjects who were not being treated for DM, the incidence of CKD was lower than for those receiving treatment. In general, 20–40% patients with type I or type II DM had a small amount of albumin in their urine after 10–15 years of stable renal function or even hyperfiltration.

Recently, the term acute kidney injury (AKI) has been applied [10]. AKI is a broad-spectrum syndrome that frequently occurs in elderly people. It is easily diagnosed by monitoring the serum creatinine levels. Female sex, age, and proteinuria are risk factors for developing advanced CKD among hospitalized AKI patients [11]. Early recognition and proper management may be useful for preventing progression to CKD. AKI is often associated with dehydration; gastrointestinal problems; cold; use of nephrotoxic drugs such as NSAIDs, contrast dye, and antibiotics; trauma; and surgery. In elderly subjects, rapid onset of AKI will not be detected if serum creatinine or urine output is not measured. In severely malnourished or emaciated subjects, eGFR based on serum creatinine may be overestimated. Also, in the elderly, there is likely a significant discrepancy between the urinary protein/creatinine ratio and daily proteinuria due to loss of muscle mass and renal function.

10.2.3 Causes of CKD Common in Elderly People

In addition to DM and hypertension (nephrosclerosis), multiple myeloma, gout, drug-induced CKD, hepatitis-associated, renal amyloidosis, and vasculitis are often seen in elderly people. Also, urologic diseases such as prostate hypertrophy in men, urinary tract stones, and malignancies of the urinary tract should be kept in mind. It is important to take the family history and query lifestyle factors, such as smoking, alcohol intake, and supplement food/pill consumption.

The Japan Renal Biopsy Registry (J-RBR) is a nationwide renal biopsy database organized by the Japanese Society of Nephrology [12]. They reported renal disease in elderly (age ≥65 years old) and very elderly (age ≥80 years old) Japanese. Compared with the control group (20–64 years of age), membranous nephropathy, MPO-ANCA-positive nephritis, and amyloid nephropathy are more common in the elderly ($P < 0.001$), and IgA nephropathy is less common ($P < 0.001$). Secular trends in the incidence of ESRD and its risk factors in Japanese patients with immunoglobulin A nephropathy were recently reported [13].

10.3 Outcomes of CKD

10.3.1 End-Stage Renal Disease (ESRD)

According to the JSDT2015 annual report, the prevalence of ESRD is 2592 per million population ($N > 320,000$) in Japan. We studied participants of the general screening program in Okinawa, Japan [14–16]. The prevalence of ESRD is more than 3000 per million population in Okinawa. Figure 10.1 shows the cumulative incidence of ESRD by age at screening in both sexes. The number of patients with ESRD is quite low among those less than 40 years of age. The incidence of ESRD increases with age, but the increase begins later for women than for men. Compared with women, men have a higher prevalence of risk factors, such as obesity, smoking, dyslipidemia, hypertension, DM, and others. Also, treatment compliance is generally not as good in men as in women.

There is no consensus regarding when to initiate dialysis therapy. The acceptance rate to begin dialysis therapy may differ among districts and countries. In Japan, the ability to begin dialysis is a luxury, and the mean eGFR at the start of dialysis must be ~6–8 mL/min/1.73 m² [3, 7]. Cases receiving optimal conservative care and no dialysis, however, are increasing. Among elderly people, it is increasingly difficult to receive regular dialysis therapy due to the lack of transportation and daily care, as well as to the presence of serious medical conditions such as cognitive dysfunction, CVD, malignancies, protein-energy wasting, and infection. Those with vascular access problems may be accepted for continuous ambulatory peritoneal dialysis.

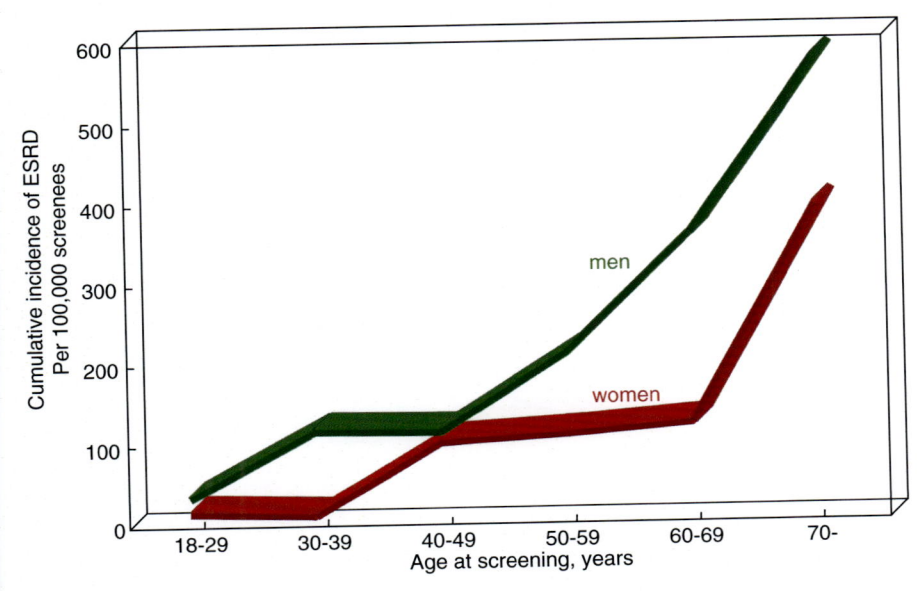

Fig. 10.1   The cumulative incidence of end-stage renal disease (ESRD) by age at screening in both sexes in Okinawa, Japan [14]

10.3.2   *Mortality Rate*

The association of age at several levels of kidney function with mortality is shown in Fig. 10.2 [17]. Among the elderly, the mortality rate increases sharply in those with a lower eGFR. The hazard ratio for death is approximately four times higher when the eGFR is 15 mL/min/1.73 m² compared with an eGFR of 95 mL/min/1.73 m². Interestingly, a high eGFR is also associated with a higher mortality rate. This finding indicates the limitation of serum creatinine-based eGFR as serum creatinine levels also reflect muscle mass.

In addition, a higher albumin-creatinine ratio (ACR) is associated with higher mortality (Fig. 10.3). An ACR ≥300 is roughly equal to dipstick protein ≥2+. Measuring the ACR is not common in Japan, except in patients with early diabetic nephropathy. A higher ACR is often associated with atherosclerotic vascular damage. If the ACR is high enough to cause nephrotic syndrome, complications such as hypoalbuminemia, hypercholesterolemia, and edema may develop.

Survival of dialysis patients is poor compared with the general population, as they have both conventional and non-conventional risk factors [18]. In general, risk of death is higher in people with either a low or high body mass index (BMI). Obesity is a risk factor for CVD and death. This is not necessarily true in patients with CKD, however, particularly dialysis patients, a phenomenon termed "reverse epidemiology" [19]. A similar phenomenon is observed with other risk factors such

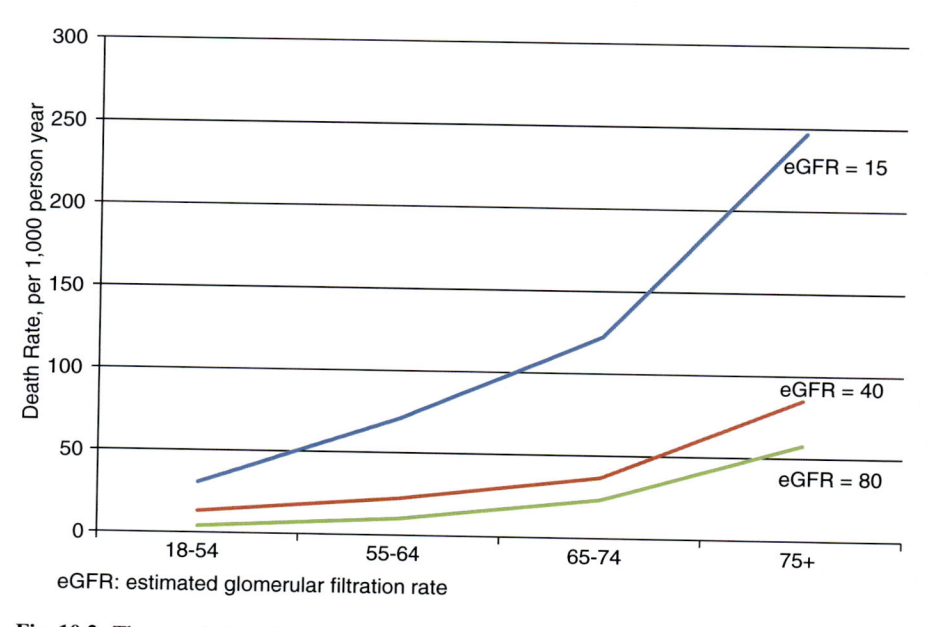

Fig. 10.2 The association of age at several levels of kidney function with death rate [17]

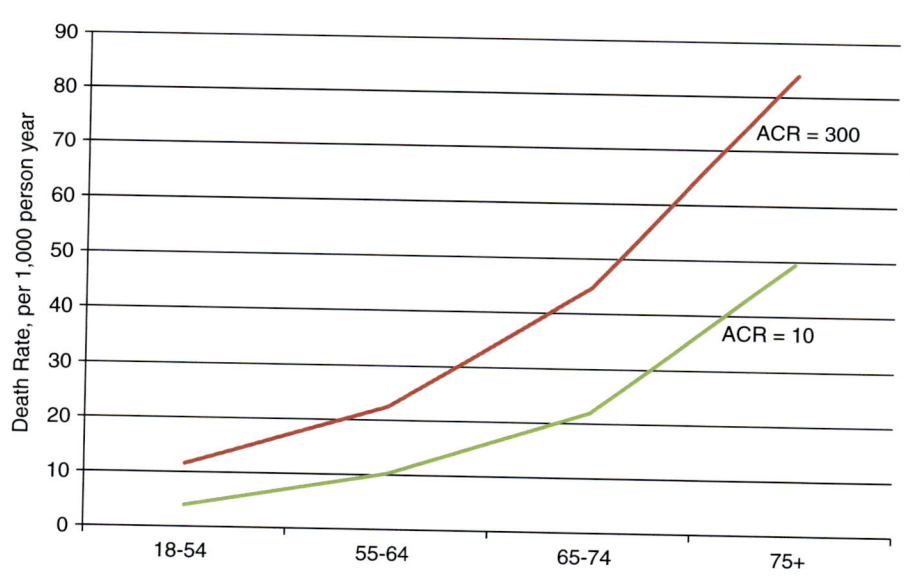

Fig. 10.3 The association of age at several levels of albumin-creatinine ratio (ACR) with death rate [17]

as serum cholesterol, blood pressure, serum creatinine, serum parathyroid hormone, serum ferritin, and calorie and/or protein intake.

10.4 Management of CKD

10.4.1 Non-dialysis-Dependent Patients

Treatment of CKD depends on the cause, such as the degree of albuminuria (proteinuria), eGFR, and associated condition. In addition to recommending a healthy lifestyle and cessation of smoking, treatment of hypertension and DM is important. Dietary instruction is similar to that for the younger generation, but the nutritional status should be carefully monitored. In particular, activities of daily living and exercise activity should be evaluated [20, 21]. Maintaining muscle mass and strength is important. The accepted frequency for monitoring in patients with advanced CKD is three times a year [20].

In Japan, we monitor patients more frequently than recommended by the Kidney Disease: Improving Global Outcomes (KDIGO) foundation. In addition to regular monitoring, support from nutritionists and other co-medical staff is helpful to prevent CKD progression [22]. Enthusiastic and professional support is mandatory to help patients adhere to lifestyle modifications and dietary instruction and clinic visits. In this regard, official and social-community support to stop smoking and restrict salt intake is underway in Japan.

Diabetes mellitus: DM (mostly type 2) is a leading cause of ESRD requiring dialysis therapy in Japan (Fig. 10.4). Although the incidence seems to have plateaued, the number remains at around 16,000 annually. The mean age at start of dialysis therapy is increasing even in DM patients. In addition to RAS inhibitors, introduction of a sodium glucose cotransporter 2 (SGLT2) inhibitor may further reduce the incidence of DM-ESRD. The adverse effects of these inhibitors are a concern, however, particularly in elderly CKD patients.

Hypertension: In elderly patients, the target blood pressure level is similar to that in younger adults [21]. Elderly patients, however, are prone to developing orthostatic hypotension, rapid changes in blood pressure, and other untoward symptoms. Restriction of salt intake with a target level of less than 5 g/day is indicated for hypertension. The use of an angiotensin receptor blocker or angiotensin-converting enzyme inhibitor is strongly recommended for DM patients with albuminuria. According to the KDIGO Blood Pressure Guideline, the target blood pressure is $\leq 140/90$ mmHg and $\leq 130/80$ mmHg if associated with microalbuminuria (>3 mg/mmol).

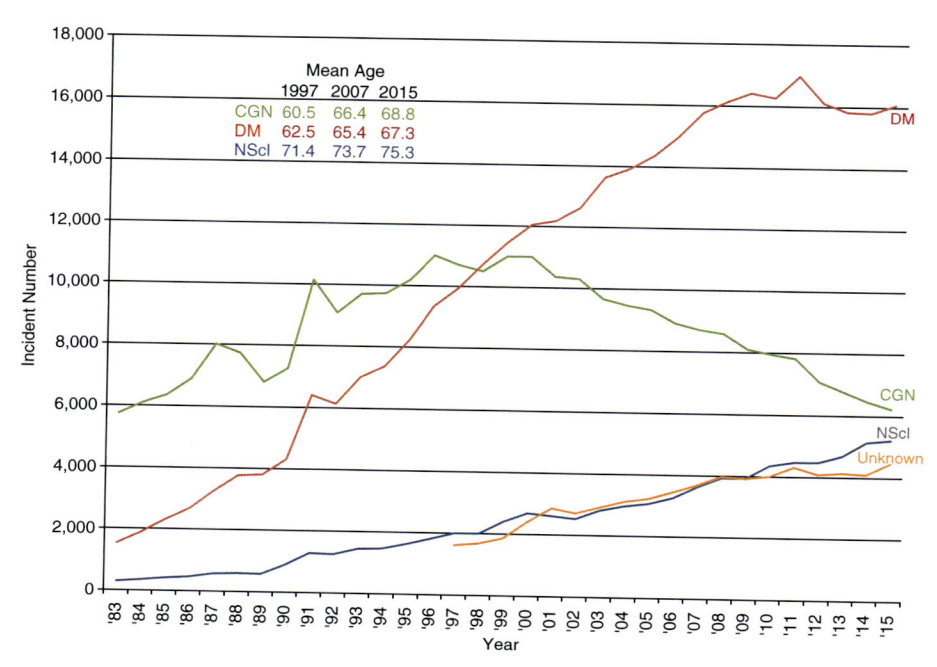

Fig. 10.4 Incident number of dialysis patients by primary renal disease in Japan from 1983 to 2015 (Data from the annual data of the Japanese Society for Dialysis Therapy). Reproduced by K. Iseki based on series of JSDT annual reports. Accessed on 30 Jan 2017 [3]

A recent SPRINT study, however, demonstrated the possible benefits of further reducing the target blood pressure [23–25]. The impact of this paper has been very strong, and the guidelines are currently under revision. Blood pressure in the SPRINT study, however, was measured using an unattended automated blood pressure device.

Renal anemia: It is common to see anemia, usually normocytic normochromic, in patients with CKD stage 3b–5. The main cause of renal anemia is deficiency of erythrocyte-stimulating hormone (erythropoietin, EPO). Several EPO drugs are available, and they are recommended to maintain hemoglobin levels at 10 g/dL and over. Many observational studies demonstrated that EPO drugs improve survival and reduce the incidence of heart failure among patients with non-dialysis-dependent CKD. Several randomized controlled trials (RCTs), however, did not reveal a benefit of EPOs to improve survival in patients with stage 5d CKD [26–28]. The reasons for this discrepancy are not yet clear.

CKD-mineral bone disorder (MBD): Bone fracture and ectopic and vascular calcifications are frequently observed in dialysis patients [29]. They are also common among patients with stage 3b–5 CKD that are not on dialysis. Regular monitoring of the serum levels of phosphate, calcium, and parathyroid hormone is mandatory as the eGFR declines. The KDIGO published guidelines regarding CKD-MBD management in 2009 [29], which were recently revised [30], but there is a paucity of well-powered trials. Guidelines for blood pressure in stage 5d CKD are still being developed.

10.4.2   Dialysis-Dependent Patients

The presence of comorbid conditions such as cardiovascular disease, malignancies, cognitive dysfunction, and protein-energy wasting [31] is increasingly recognized among elderly incident dialysis patients. Survival of those with such comorbid conditions is poor. After acceptance for chronic dialysis therapy, it is important to take in an adequate amount of calories, protein, and exercise, supported by regular dialysis therapy. The JSDT recommends prescribing "conventional dialysis," which denotes hemodialysis for at least 4 h three times per week.

In Japan, we recommend creating an arteriovenous fistula before the initiation of dialysis therapy. The most common blood flow rate is about 200 mL/min. Unfortunately, guidelines for dialysis initiation and management of dialysis patients are lacking due to paucity of well-powered trials. Several randomized controlled trials using statins and EPO-stimulating agents revealed no clinical benefits among dialysis patients. Reasons for the failure of these trials could explain the complex nature of dialysis patients. These patients may have a large number of risk factors, including comorbid conditions, dialysis prescription, and a variety of socioeconomic backgrounds. Quality of life and survival are widely distributed among the dialysis population.

10.4.3   Transplant Patients

The Organ Transplant Act was enforced in October 1997, in Japan. The number of cadaveric renal transplantations has not rapidly increased and has rather remained low with the highest number being 112 in 2011. The number is stable at around 80–100 per year.

As shown in Fig. 10.4, ESRD due to chronic glomerulonephritis is decreasing, and the mean age at the start of dialysis is increasing. The number of preemptive kidney transplantations has recently begun to increase, as the recipients would rather not begin dialysis therapy. Most of the donors are spouses and require careful follow-up after donation [32].

10.5   Perspectives

10.5.1   Paucity of Trials in Nephrology

The incidence of ESRD and death is not frequent, and a large number of subjects and long-term observations are required; therefore, it is difficult to obtain financial support for these studies. CKD patients are excluded from many RCTs. The incidence of ESRD and deaths is used as an outcome of the study. Doubling of the serum creatinine level equal to a 57% reduction in eGFR over 2 years has also been used as a surrogate marker of ESRD and death. We tested the rate of decline of eGFR as a surrogate marker of CKD outcome among Japanese. We confirmed that a 30% decline in eGFR over 2 years could be a useful surrogate marker for predicting ESRD [33]. Also, we evaluated the significance of changes in dipstick proteinuria [34]. Therefore, we are expecting an increase in drug trials in the field of nephrology [35].

10.5.2 Specific Health Check Program (SHCP)

In Japan, the SHCP was started in 2008 to reduce the socioeconomic burden related to metabolic syndrome and obesity [36, 37]. The target was people aged 40–74 years. We have performed cross-sectional, longitudinal, and outcome (using national death certificate) studies using the SHCP database. In the cross-sectional study, lifestyle factors such as smoking, alcohol intake, exercise, dietary habits, and non-restorative sleep were significantly associated with CKD prevalence [38]. Moreover, modifications of these lifestyle factors decreased the incidence of proteinuria [39]. Unfortunately, the SHCP has no data for people aged 75 years and over. We expect that our observational studies will provide a basis for better understanding lifestyle-related diseases among the Japanese.

We also analyzed the impact of CKD screening on the medical budget. To prevent the rise in medical and dialysis costs, early detection and lifestyle interventions are helpful. In this regard, we demonstrated that dipstick proteinuria tests and measurements of serum creatinine are a cost-effective strategy for CKD [40–42]. CKD is usually asymptomatic in its early stage (1–3a), and therefore efforts to publicize the dangers of CKD are important. In this regard, World Kidney Day, which is held on the second Thursday of March every year, should be helpful for educating the population on the dangers of CKD.

10.5.3 KDIGO

KDIGO is an international organization whose mission is to improve the care and outcomes of CKD patients worldwide by promoting the coordination, collaboration, and integration of initiatives to develop and implement clinical practice guidelines (CPGs). The number of patients requiring kidney replacement therapy has increased dramatically throughout the world over the last four decades. Some contributing factors include improved survival of the general population, an increased incidence of CKD, changes in universal availability of dialysis in various countries, and significant broadening of the kidney replacement therapy acceptance criteria. As a result, kidney replacement therapy has become available to increasing numbers of older patients with multiple comorbid illnesses such as DM and congestive heart failure. KDIGO has published 11 CPGs and held 34 Controversies Conferences in various fields of nephrology. CPGs are based on the evidence, such as RCTs, and expert opinions. Unfortunately, patients with CKD and elderly people have been excluded from RCTs. This was probably related to the lack of an adequate surrogate marker other than doubling the serum creatinine. Doubling the serum creatinine is equal to a 57% decline in eGFR over 2 years and has been used as a surrogate of hard outcomes. Adopting hard outcomes such as death or initiation of dialysis may not be feasible for RCTs among elderly CKD patients. Instead, a slower decline in eGFR, such as a 30–40% decline over 2 years, is a useful surrogate marker to examine ESRD incidence.

KDIGO published CPGs for the Evaluation and Management of Chronic Kidney Disease in 2013 [20]. They provided an update of the 2002 KDOQI Clinical Practice Guidelines for Chronic Kidney Disease: Evaluation, Classification, and Stratification following a decade of focused research and clinical practice in CKD. Specifically, the guidelines retained the definition of CKD but presented an enhanced classification framework for CKD, elaborating on the identification and prognosis of CKD. Several complications related to CKD have been discussed such as anemia, blood pressure, mineral and CKD-MBD, lipids, and so on. The Controversies Conferences were held prior to the development and implementation of the guidelines.

10.5.4 Dementia

Dementia has become a priority worldwide in terms of both public health and social care due to its rapidly increasing burden on communities. The increased incidence and improved survival rate of patients with Alzheimer's disease has resulted in a steep increase in the prevalence of Alzheimer's disease among the Japanese elderly [43]. Whether or not uremic toxin(s) per se play a role in dementia is controversial, but dementia is prevalent among the chronic dialysis population. Once patients accepted for chronic dialysis treatment develop dementia, it becomes very difficult to continue the treatment. The JSDT proposed a shared decision-making process regarding the initiation and continuation of maintenance hemodialysis for patients with dementia [44].

10.6 Conclusion

The elderly population is rapidly increasing in both developed and developing countries, and Japan has the highest rate of increase. The screening system for CKD is highly developed in Japan and begins with school children through the general population. The decreasing incidence of ESRD due to chronic glomerulonephritis may be explained by this health screening system and socioeconomic environment. ESRD due to DM and nephrosclerosis due to hypertension, however, is increasing.

Signs and symptoms associated with normal aging may, at least partly, be explained by the physiologic decline in the GFR. Therefore, the clinical relevance of CKD among the elderly population is becoming more evident. More studies of patient reported outcomes are needed for the development of CPGs.

References

1. Levey A, de Jong PE, Coresh J, et al. Chronic kidney disease—definition, classification and prognosis: a KDIGO controversies conference report. Kidney Int. 2011;80:17–28.
2. Sarnak MJ, Levey AS, Schoolwerth AC, et al. Kidney disease as a risk factor for development of cardiovascular disease. A statement from the American Heart Association Councils on kidney in cardiovascular disease, high blood pressure research, clinical cardiology, and epidemiology and prevention. Circulation. 2003;108:2154–69.
3. The Japanese Society for Dialysis Therapy. JSDT annual reports. http://www.jsdt.or.jp/. Accessed 30 Jan 2017.
4. Matsuo S, Imai E, Horio M, et al. Revised equations for estimated GFR from serum creatinine in Japan. Am J Kidney Dis. 2009;53(6):982–92.
5. Imai E, Horio M, Iseki K, et al. Prevalence of chronic kidney disease (CKD) in the Japanese general population predicted by MDRD equation modified by a Japanese coefficient. Clin Exp Nephrol. 2007;11:156–63.
6. Imai E, Horio M, Yamagata K, et al. Slower decline of glomerular filtration rate in the Japanese general population: a longitudinal 10-year follow-up study. Hypertens Res. 2008;31(3):433–41.
7. Watanabe Y, Yamagata K, Nishi S, et al. JSDT clinical guideline for "hemodialysis initiation for maintenance hemodialysis". Ther Apher Dial. 2015;19(Suppl 1):93–107.
8. Yamagata K, Ishida K, Sairenchi T, et al. Risk factors for chronic kidney disease in a community-based population: a 10-year follow-up study. Kidney Int. 2007;71:159–66.
9. Tozawa M, Iseki K, Iseki C, et al. Influence of smoking and obesity on the development of proteinuria. Kidney Int. 2002;62:956–62.
10. Okusa MD, Davenport A. Reading between the (guide) lines—the KDIGO practice guideline on acute kidney injury in the individual patient. Kidney Int. 2014;85(1):39–48.
11. James MT, Pannu N, Hemmelgarn BR, et al. Derivation and external validation of prediction models for advanced chronic kidney disease following acute kidney injury. JAMA. 2017;318(18):1787–97.
12. Yokoyama H, Sugiyama H, Sato H, et al. Renal disease in the elderly and the very elderly Japanese: analysis of the Japan Renal Biopsy Registry (J-RBR). Clin Exp Nephrol. 2012;16:903–20.
13. Tanaka S, Ninomiya T, Katafuchi R, et al. Secular trends in the incidence of end-stage renal disease and its risk factors in Japanese patients with immunoglobulin A nephropathy. Nephrol Dial Transplant. 2018;33(6):963–71.
14. Iseki K, Iseki C, Ikemiya Y, Fukiyama K. Risk of developing end-stage renal disease in a cohort of mass screening. Kidney Int. 1996;49:800–5.
15. Iseki K. Factors influencing development of end-stage renal disease. Clin Exp Nephrol. 2005;9:5–14.
16. Iseki K. Proteinuria as a predictor of rapid eGFR decline. Nat Rev Nephrol. 2013;9:570–1.
17. Hallan SI, Matsushita K, Sang Y, et al. Age and association of kidney measures with mortality and end-stage renal disease. JAMA. 2012;308(22):2349–60.
18. Iseki K, Shinzato T, Nagura Y, Akiba T. Factors influencing long-term survival in patients on chronic dialysis. Clin Exp Nephrol. 2004;8:89–97.
19. Kalantar-Zadeh K, Block G, Humphreys MH, Kopple JD. Reverse epidemiology of cardiovascular risk factors in maintenance dialysis patients. Kidney Int. 2003;63:793–808.

20. Kidney Disease: Improving Global Outcomes (KDIGO) CKD Work Group. KDIGO 2012 clinical practice guideline for the evaluation and management of chronic kidney disease. Kidney Int Suppl. 2013;3:1–150.
21. Kidney Disease: Improving Global Outcomes (KDIGO) Blood Pressure Work Group. KDIGO clinical practice guideline for the management of blood pressure in chronic kidney disease. Kidney Int Suppl. 2012;2:337–414.
22. Yamagata K, Makino H, Iseki K, et al. Effect of behavior modification on outcome in early- to moderate-stage chronic kidney disease: a cluster-randomized trial. PLoS One. 2016;11(3):e0151422.
23. Williamson JD, Supiano MA, Applegate WB, et al. Intensive vs standard blood pressure control and cardiovascular disease outcomes in adults aged ≥75 years a randomized clinical trial. JAMA. 2016;315(24):2673–82.
24. Chobanian IV. SPRINT results in older patients—how low to go? JAMA. 2016;315(24):2669–70.
25. Sexton DJ, Canney M, O'Connell MDL, et al. Injurious falls and syncope in older community-dwelling adults meeting inclusion criteria for SPRINT. JAMA Intern Med. 2017;177(9):1385–7.
26. Besarab A, Bolton WK, Browne JK, et al. The effects of normal as compared with low hematocrit values in patients with cardiac disease who are receiving hemodialysis and epoetin. N Engl J Med. 1998;339:584–90.
27. Palmer SC, Navaneethan SD, Craig JC, et al. Meta-analysis: erythropoiesis-stimulating agents in patients with chronic kidney disease. Ann Intern Med. 2010;153:23–33.
28. Kidney Disease: Improving Global Outcomes (KDIGO) Anemia Work Group. KDIGO clinical practice guideline for anemia in chronic kidney disease. Kidney Int Suppl. 2012;2:279–335.
29. Kidney Disease: Improving Global Outcomes (KDIGO) CKD-MBD Work Group. KDIGO clinical practice guideline for the diagnosis, evaluation, prevention, and treatment of chronic kidney disease-mineral and bone disorder (CKD-MBD). Kidney Int Suppl. 2009;113: S1–130.
30. Kidney Disease: Improving Global Outcomes (KDIGO) CKD-MBD Update Work Group. KDIGO 2017 clinical practice guideline update for the diagnosis, evaluation, prevention, and treatment of CKD-MBD. Kidney Int Suppl. 2017;7:1–59.
31. Ikizler TA, Cano NJ, Franch H, et al. Prevention and treatment of protein energy wasting in chronic kidney disease patients: a consensus statement by the International Society of Renal Nutrition and Metabolism. Kidney Int. 2013;84(6):1096–107.
32. Lentine KL, Kasiske BL, Levey AS, et al. KDIGO clinical practice guideline on the evaluation and care of living kidney donors. Transplantation. 2017;101(8S Suppl 1):S1–S109.
33. Kanda E, Usui T, Kashihara N, et al. Importance of glomerular filtration rate change as surrogate endpoint for the future incidence of end-stage renal disease in general Japanese population: community-based cohort study. Clin Exp Nephrol. 2018;22(2):318–27.
34. Usui T, Kanda E, Iseki C, et al. Observation period for changes in proteinuria and risk prediction of end-stage renal disease in general population. Nephrology. 2018 (in press).
35. Strippoli GFM, Craig JC, Schena FP. The number, quality, and coverage of randomized controlled trials in nephrology. JASN. 2004;15:411–9.
36. Iseki K, Asahi K, Moriyama T, et al. Risk factor profiles based on eGFR and dipstick proteinuria: analysis of the participants of the specific health check and guidance system in Japan 2008. Clin Exp Nephrol. 2012;16:244–9.
37. Iseki K, Asahi K, Yamagata K, et al. Mortality risk among screened subjects of the specific health check and guidance program in Japan 2008–2012. Clin Exp Nephrol. 2017;21: 978–85.
38. Wakasugi M, Kazama JJ, Narita I, et al. Associations between combined lifestyle factors and non-restorative sleep in Japan: a cross-sectional study based on a Japanese health database. PLoS One. 2014;9(9):e108718.
39. Wakasugi M, Kazama JJ, Narita I, et al. Association between overall lifestyle changes and incidence of proteinuria: a population-based, cohort study. Intern Med. 2017;56(12):1475–84.
40. Kondo M, Yamagata K, Hoshi SL, et al. Cost-effectiveness of chronic kidney disease mass screening test in Japan. Clin Exp Nephrol. 2012;16:279–91.

41. Kondo M, Yamagata K, Hoshi SL, et al. Budget impact analysis of chronic kidney disease mass screening test in Japan. Clin Exp Nephrol. 2014;18(6):885–91.
42. Iseki K, Iseki C, Kurahashi I, Watanabe T. Effect of glomerular filtration rate and proteinuria on medical cost among screened subjects. Clin Exp Nephrol. 2013;17:372–8.
43. Ohara T, Hata J, Yoshida D, et al. Trends in dementia prevalence, incidence, and survival rate in a Japanese community. Neurology. 2017;88(20):1925–32.
44. Watanabe Y, Hirakata H, Okada K, et al. Proposal for the shared decision-making process regarding initiation and continuation of maintenance hemodialysis. Ther Apher Dial. 2015;19(Suppl 1):108–17.

Chapter 11
Lung Cancer in the Elderly: The Most Dominant Cause of Cancer Death in Japan

Chikako Kiyohara, Yoichi Nakanishi, and Masakazu Washio

Abstract Lung cancer is a major cause of cancer-related death in Japan, and the overall survival rate was still poor. The majority of individuals diagnosed with lung cancer are elderly people aged $\geq$65 years. Although chronic inhalation of cigarette smoke is a major risk factor to the development of lung cancer, genetic factors have been implicated to account for some of the observed differences in lung cancer susceptibility. A number of studies have examined lung cancer susceptibility based on the presence of high-frequency, low-penetrance genetic polymorphisms. As exposure to harmful chemicals or reactive oxygen species via cigarette smoking is thought to contribute to the development of lung cancer, genetic polymorphisms involved in xenobiotic metabolism, DNA repair, and inflammation might be promising candidates. In order to evaluate whether the impact of genetic polymorphisms on lung cancer differs between elderly and younger people, we evaluated potential 31 genetic polymorphisms in a stratified analysis by age category (aged $\geq$65 and <65 years). Seven polymorphisms, namely, *CYP1A1* rs4646903, *CYP1A1* rs1048943, *GSTM1* deletion, *GSTP1* rs1695, *SULTA1* rs9282861, *TP53BP1* rs560191, and *CRP* rs2794520, were associated with lung cancer risk in the elderly. However, there was little difference in the impact of polymorphism on lung cancer risk between the elderly and non-elderly groups. In this chapter, we would like to discuss the importance of the prevention of smoking (the best established and strongest avoidable risk factor) at early age for successful aging.

C. Kiyohara (✉)
Department of Preventive Medicine, Graduate School of Medical Sciences, Kyushu University, Fukuoka City, Fukuoka, Japan
e-mail: chikako@phealth.med.kyushu-u.ac.jp

Y. Nakanishi
Research Institute for Diseases of the Chest, Graduate School of Medical Sciences, Kyushu University, Fukuoka City, Fukuoka, Japan

M. Washio
Department of Community Health and Clinical Epidemiology, St. Mary's College, Kurume City, Fukuoka, Japan
e-mail: washiomasa@yahoo.co.jp

© Springer Nature Singapore Pte Ltd. 2019
M. Washio, C. Kiyohara (eds.), *Health Issues and Care System for the Elderly*, Current Topics in Environmental Health and Preventive Medicine, https://doi.org/10.1007/978-981-13-1762-0_11

Keywords Cigarette smoking · DNA repair · Inflammation · Lung cancer · Metabolism · Genetic polymorphism

11.1 Introduction

Improvement of public health and advances in medicine after World War II have given Japan one of the highest average life expectancies in the world (i.e., 81.0 years old for men and 87.1 years old for women in 2016), and the proportion of the elderly (people aged ≥65 years) increased from 4.9% in 1950 to 27.3% in 2016 [1]. Increased life expectancy means the increased number of the elderly who need medical care.

Tobacco smoking is the largest single recognized cause of human cancer in Western countries [2]. Cigarette smoking alone account for about 30% of all cancer deaths in the United States and an estimated 16% of all cancers worldwide [2]. Tobacco smoking is associated with an increased risk of malignancies of both organs in direct contact with smoke, such as the esophagus and lung, and organs not in direct contact with smoke, such as the kidneys [3].

As shown in Table 11.1, cancer has been the leading cause of death in Japan since 1981 and is the major causes of death for over three decades in Japan [1]. Cerebrovascular diseases (CVD) were the leading cause of death for three decades before 1980. Heart disease deaths outnumbered CVD deaths for 1985–2016 except for the period from 1995 to 1996. Infectious diseases [tuberculosis (predominantly lung tuberculosis), pneumonia, bronchitis, gastroenteritis] were the major cause of death in Japan before 1950. As of 2016, lung cancer is the first cause of cancer death for men and the second cause of cancer death for women in an all Japanese population [1]. Table 11.2 illustrates that lung cancer mortality rate among men (242.4 per 100,000) is also the highest among all site-specific cancer death rates in the elderly (people aged ≥65 years) in Japan [1].

Lung cancer has become the most frequent malignant neoplasm among men in most countries, and a parallel increase in incidence is seen among women in Western countries although lung cancer was a rare disease before the beginning of the twentieth century [4]. As shown in Table 11.3, tobacco smoking increases the risk of lung cancer, while a diet rich in fruits and vegetables has a protective effect against lung cancer [4–6]. Washio et al. [7] conducted a case-control study in Hokkaido, Northern Japan, and found that current smokers (vs. non-smokers, odds ratio (OR) = 4.65, 95% confidence intervals (CI) = 2.17–9.97) and old age (65 years old and over vs. 40–64 years old, OR = 2.31, 95% CI = 1.41–3.80) increased the risk of lung cancer, and short sleeping time (5 h/day or less vs. 6 h/day or more, OR = 2.47, 95% CI = 0.97–6.32) showed a non-significantly increased lung cancer risk after controlling age, sex, and smoking status [7]. On the other hand, never smokers (vs. ex-smokers, OR = 0.28, 95% CI = 0.14–0.56), high intake of green tea (7 cups/day and over vs. 0–6 cups/day, OR = 0.38, 95% CI = 0.14–0.995), and frequent consumption of green and yel-

Table 11.1 Trends in causes of death between 1899 and 2016[a] [1]

	Top	Second	Third	Fourth	Fifth
1899	Pneumonia and bronchitis	CVD	All tuberculosis	Gastroenteritis	Senility[b]
1930	Gastroenteritis	Pneumonia and bronchitis	All tuberculosis	CVD	Senility[b]
1940	All tuberculosis	Pneumonia and bronchitis	CVD	Gastroenteritis	Senility[b]
1950	All tuberculosis	CVD	Pneumonia and bronchitis	Gastroenteritis	Cancers
1960	CVD	Cancers	Heart diseases	Senility[b]	Pneumonia and bronchitis
1970–1972	CVD	Cancers	Heart diseases	Accidents[c]	Senility
1973–1974	CVD	Cancers	Heart diseases	Accidents[c]	Pneumonia and bronchitis
1975–1978	CVD	Cancers	Heart diseases	Pneumonia and bronchitis	Accidents[c]
1979–1980	CVD	Cancers	Heart diseases	Pneumonia and bronchitis	Senility[a]
1981	Cancers	CVD	Heart diseases	Pneumonia and bronchitis	Senility[a]
1982–1984	Cancers	CVD	Heart diseases	Pneumonia and bronchitis	Accidents[c]
1985–1994	Cancers	Heart diseases	CVD	Pneumonia and bronchitis	Accidents[c]
1995–1996	Cancers	CVD	Heart diseases[d]	Pneumonia	Accidents
1997–2008	Cancers	Heart diseases[d]	CVD	Pneumonia	Accidents
2009–2010	Cancers	Heart diseases[d]	CVD	Pneumonia	Senility
2011	Cancers	Heart diseases[d]	Pneumonia	CVD	Accidents
2012–2016	Cancers	Heart diseases[d]	Pneumonia	CVD	Senility

CVD cerebrovascular diseases
[a]Okinawa Prefecture is not included for 1947–1973
[b]Senility without mention of psychosis
[c]Accidents and adverse effects
[d]Heart diseases without hypertensive heart diseases

low vegetables (4 days/week vs. 0–3 days/week, OR = 0.46, 95% CI = 0.26–0.81) reduced the risk of lung cancer after controlling age, sex, and smoking status [5].

Since our health status in the later life is influenced by the life experience throughout life, health promotion from pregnancy and childhood to old age is important to avoid unhealthy aging. We should remember not only tobacco smoking but also exposure to environmental tobacco smoke increases the risk of cancer [5].

Table 11.2 Site-specific cancer mortality rate per 100,000[a] in 2016

	Population aged ≥65 years			Population aged <65 years		
	Both sexes	Men	Women	Both sexes	Men	Women
Top	Lung (149.2)	Lung (242.4)	Colorectal (83.11)	Lung (24.08)	Lung (34.37)	Colorectal (14.90)
Second	Colorectal (98.78)	Stomach (135.8)	Lung (77.80)	Colorectal (17.25)	Stomach (20.29)	Breast (14.78)
Third	Stomach (91.02)	Colorectal (119.3)	Pancreas (59.27)	Stomach (15.21)	Colorectal (19.54)	Lung (13.53)
Fourth	Pancreas (66.50)	Liver (81.07)	Stomach (56.76)	Pancreas (11.34)	Liver (13.58)	Pancreas (10.54)
Fifth	Liver (55.40)	Pancreas (75.94)	Breast (35.15)	Liver (10.14)	Pancreas (12.12)	Stomach (9.999)

[a]Calculated based on the database of Vital Statistics in Japan, 2016 [1]

Table 11.3 Risk factors other than genetic factors for lung cancer in Japan and worldwide [4–6]

	Japan		Worldwide	
Factors	Association	Direction of risk	Association	Direction of risk
Smoking	Convincing	Increase	Convincing[a]	Increase
Exposure to ETS	Convincing	Increase	Convincing[a]	Increase
β-Carotene supplement	Not available		Convincing	Increase[b]
Fruits	Possible	Decrease	Probable	Decrease
Vegetables	Limited (no conclusion)		Limited (suggestive)	Decrease[c]
Physical activity	Limited (no conclusion)		Limited (suggestive)	Decrease
Alcohol use	Limited (no conclusion)		Limited (no conclusion)	

ETS environmental tobacco smoke
[a]The panel emphasizes the importance of not smoking and avoiding exposure to environmental tobacco smoke although the WCRF/AICR report would not judge the evidence on active smoking and exposure to environmental tobacco smoke
[b]Among current smokers
[c]Non-starchy vegetables

11.2   Case-Control Study to Investigate Association Between Genetic Polymorphism and Lung Cancer Risk

11.2.1   Background

Although tobacco smoking is a convincing risk factor for lung cancer, approximately one in ten smokers develops lung cancer in their lifetime indicating an inter-individual variation in susceptibility to tobacco smoking [8]. Individuals may have a unique combination of polymorphic traits that modify genetic susceptibility and response to tobacco smoking. Chemical substances in tobacco smoke must be metabolically activated to exert their noxious effects by phase I enzymes, but this is counteracted by the ongoing detoxification of activated substances (carcinogens in most situations) by phase II enzymes. Therefore, DNA damage itself is a balance between phase I and II metabolic enzymes, many of which are polymorphic. The capacity to repair DNA damage induced by activated carcinogens is also a genetic factor that may affect lung cancer risk. Furthermore, exposure to reactive oxygen species (ROS) via cigarette smoking is thought to contribute to the development of lung cancer [9]. Phase I enzymes contribute to the formation of ROS, whereas phase II enzymes play a critical role in the detoxification and reduction of ROS [10]. Chronic inflammation has been implicated in the development of several human malignancies, including lung cancer [11]. Pulmonary inflammation may promote tumor formation by the generation of ROS and secretion of cytokines, chemokines, and pro-angiogenic factors [12]. Lung cancer susceptibility may be associated with genetic polymorphisms involved in the inflammatory response.

The primary advantage of genetic markers is to allow the identification of a high-risk group for lung cancer and guide individualized therapy. Thus, reliable genetic markers for lung cancer are urgently required. It has been hypothesized that the rise in cancer diagnosis for elderly persons may be due to DNA damage by ROS [13]. In this chapter, we reanalyzed the data from our case-control studies [14–21] limited to elderly people aged 65 years and over, with special reference to genetic polymorphisms involved in xenobiotic metabolism, DNA repair, and inflammation. For comparison, the same polymorphisms among the non-elderly population (<65 years) were determined.

11.2.2 Materials and Methods

11.2.2.1 Study Subjects and Data Collection

Lung cancer patients were enrolled in Kyushu University Hospital (Research Institute for Diseases of the Chest, Kyushu University) and its collaborating hospitals. The suitable cases ($n = 462$) were patients with primary lung cancer that were newly diagnosed and histologically confirmed during the period from 1996 to 2008. The participation rate among the cases was 100%. Histological types were categorized into four major types according to the International Classification of Diseases for Oncology (ICD-O), second edition: adenocarcinoma (8140, 8211, 8230–8231, 8250–8260, 8323, 8480–8490, 8550–8560, 8570–8572), squamous cell carcinoma (8050–8076), small cell carcinoma (8040–8045), and large cell carcinoma (8012–8031, 8310). Controls ($n = 379$) were the hospitalized patients without clinical history of any type of malignancy, ischemic heart disease, or chronic respiratory disease during the same period. Controls were not, individually or in larger groups, matched to cases. Controls were approached by their attending physicians to be recruited as control subjects. None of the controls refused to participate in this study. A self-administered questionnaire was used to collect data on demographic and lifestyle factors such as age, years of education, smoking, alcohol consumption, environmental tobacco exposure from spouse, etc. All subjects were unrelated ethnic Japanese. The details have been described elsewhere [14–21]. The study subjects were stratified by age group, namely, the elderly group (people aged ≥65 years, 303 cases and 114 controls) and the non-elderly group (people aged <65 years, 159 cases and 265 controls). A total of 462 cases and 379 controls were included in this analysis.

The study protocol was approved by our institutional review board, and all participants were provided written informed consent.

11.2.2.2   Genetic Analysis

Genomic DNA was extracted from blood samples. Genotyping of 31 polymorphisms (xenobiotic metabolism, *CYP1A1* rs464903, *CYP1A1* rs1048943, *CYP1A2* rs76551, *CYP1A2* rs2069514, *CYP2A6* deletion, *CYP2A13* rs8192789, *CYP2E1* rs2031920, *MPO* rs2333227, *GSTM1* deletion, *GSTT1* deletion, *GSTP1* rs1695, *NQO1* rs1800566, *SULT1A1* rs9282861, *NAT2* genotypes determined by *NAT2*4*, *5B*, *6A*, or *7B* allele; DNA repair, *ERCC2* rs13181, *XRCC1* rs25487, *AXRCC3* rs861539, *OGG1* rs1052113, *TP53* rs1042522, *TP53BP1* rs560191; and inflammation, *IL1B1* rs1143634, *IL6* rs1800796, *IL8* rs4073, *IL10* rs180871, *IL13* rs1800925, *CRP* rs2794520, *NOS2* rs2297518, *CYBA* rs4673, *TNFA* rs1799724, *TNFRA2* rs1061622, *NFkB* rs283649) was conducted with blinding to case-control status. The details of the methods have been described elsewhere [14–21]. For quality control, both assays were repeated on a random 5% of all samples, and the replicates were 100% concordant.

11.2.2.3   Statistical Analysis

Comparisons of means, proportions, and medians were based on the unpaired t test, χ^2 test, and Wilcoxon rank-sum test, respectively. The distribution of the genotypes of polymorphisms in controls was compared with that expected from Hardy-Weinberg equilibrium (HWE) by the chi-square (Pearson) test. Unconditional logistic regression was used to compute the ORs and their 95% CIs, with adjustments for several covariates. Subjects were considered current smokers if they smoked or stopped smoking less than 1 year before either the date of diagnosis of lung cancer or the date of completion of the questionnaires (controls). Never smokers were defined as those who had never smoked in their lifetime. Former smokers were those who had stopped smoking 1 or more years before either the date of diagnosis of lung cancer or the date of completion of the questionnaires (controls).

Based on "Healthy Japan 21" (National Health Promotion in the twenty-first century), heavy drinkers were defined as those who drank more than 60 g of alcohol per day. As "Healthy Japan 21" has emphasized drinking an appropriate volume of alcohol (20 g of alcohol per day), appropriate drinkers were defined as those who did not exceed 20 g of alcohol intake per day. The appropriate volume of alcohol use may have a protective effect on life expectancy and morbidity [22]. Unlike cigarette smoke, ingested alcohol is eliminated from the body by various metabolic mechanisms, and the alcohol elimination process begins almost immediately. Significant relationships between excessive drinking and lung cancer have been reported, while appropriate drinking has not shown the same effects [23]. In terms of alcohol consumption, the subjects were classified into the following three groups based on their intake for at least 1 year: those who drank more than 60 g of alcohol per day (heavy drinkers), those who drank more than 20 g of alcohol per day but not exceeding 60 g per day (moderate drinkers), and those who drank less than 20 g of alcohol per day (appropriate drinkers). Appropriate drinkers included infrequent and nondrinkers because the lung cancer risks were comparable among them [17].

Genotype impact was assessed by a score test for each genotype as follows: (0) homozygous for the major allele, (1) heterozygous, and (2) homozygous for the minor allele. All statistical analyses were performed using the computer program STATA Version 14.2 (STATA Corporation, College Station, TX). All P values were two-sided, with those less than 0.05 considered statistically significant.

11.2.3   Results

11.2.3.1   Characteristics of Study Subjects

Table 11.4 summarizes the distributions of selected characteristics among subjects [14–21]. As controls were not selected to match lung cancer patients on age and sex, there were significant differences in age ($P < 0.001$) between lung cancer patients and controls in both the elderly and non-elderly groups. Sex ratio was significantly different between cases and controls in the non-elderly group ($P = 0.001$). Compared with control subjects, lung cancer patients were more likely to report a history of smoking in the both groups ($P < 0.001$). Pack-years of smoking were significantly different between cases and controls in the two groups. We excluded pack-years (the number of packs of cigarettes smoked/day multiplied by years of smoking) from the logistic models because of high correlation with age (avoiding the problem of potential collinearity). Compared with control subjects, lung cancer patients were more likely to report a history of alcohol drinking in the non-elderly group ($P = 0.001$).

11.2.3.2   Association Between Genetic Polymorphisms Involved in Xenobiotic Metabolism and Lung Cancer Risk

The genotype frequencies of 14 polymorphisms were consistent with Hardy-Weinberg equilibrium (HWE) among controls, except for *CYP2E1* rs2031920 ($P = 0.016$) in the elderly group (data not shown). As shown in Table 11.5 [14, 15,

Table 11.4 Selected characteristics of lung cancer cases and controls [14–21]

Characteristics	Aged ≥65 years			Aged <65 years		
	Cases (n = 303)	Controls (n = 114)	P	Cases (n = 159)	Controls (n = 265)	P
Age (year), mean (95% CI)	71.4 (70.9–71.8)	69.4 (68.8–70.0)	<0.001	56.0 (54.9–57.1)	50.1 (48.7–51.4)	<0.001
Sex, n (%)						
Male	191 (63.0)	82 (71.9)		96 (60.4)	201 (75.9)	
Female	112 (37.0)	32 (28.1)	0.089	63 (39.6)	64 (24.2)	0.001
Smoking status, n (%)						
Current smoker	128 (42.2)	38 (33.3)		70 (44.0)	91 (34.3)	
Former smoker	72 (23.8)	13 (11.4)		39 (24.5)	28 (10.6)	
Never smoker	103 (34.0)	63 (55.3)	<0.001	50 (31.5)	146 (55.1)	<0.001
Ever-smoker[a]	200 (66.0)	51 (44.7)	<0.001	109 (68.6)	119 (44.9)	<0.001
Pack-years among ever-smokers, mean (95% CI)	58.7 (54.8–62.5)	48.4 (43.9–52.9)	0.011	46.5 (41.6–51.5)	30.3 (27.2–33.5)	<0.001
Drinking status, n (%)						
Non drinker	120 (39.6)	58 (50.9)		58 (36.5)	146 (55.1)	
Moderate drinker[b]	85 (28.1)	27 (23.7)		45 (28.3)	57 (21.5)	
Excessive drinker[c]	98 (32.3)	29 (25.4)	0.114	56 (35.2)	62 (23.4)	0.001
Exposure to ETS among never smokers, n (%)						
Positive	60 (58.3)	34 (54.0)	0.589	39 (78.0)	101 (69.2)	0.233
Education (year), mean (95% CI)	13.4 (13.2–13.6)	13.7 (13.3–14.1)	0.270	15.1 (14.7–15.5)	15.4 (15.1–15.6)	0.173

ETS environmental tobacco smoke, *CI* confidence interval

[a]Current and former smokers were combined (ever-smokers)

[b]Subjects who drink more than 0 and less than 20 g of alcohol per day

[c]Subjects who drink more than 20 g of alcohol per day

18, 20, 24, 25], the minor homozygotes of *CYP1A1* rs4646903 (OR = 2.36, 95% CI = 1.13–4.94) were significantly associated with an increased lung cancer risk even after adjustment for age, sex, education, smoking status, and drinking status. With the increasing number of the C allele, there was a significant trend of higher risk of lung cancer (P_{trend} = 0.019). The null genotype of the *GSTM1* deletion polymorphism was at a 1.61-fold (95% CI = 1.01–2.55) increased risk of lung cancer. *CYP1A1* rs1048943 (OR = 1.64, 95% CI = 1.03–2.62), *GSTP1* rs1695 (OR = 2.25, 95% CI = 1.29–3.92), and *SULT1A1* rs9282861 (OR = 1.64, 95% CI = 1.001–2.69) were associated with lung cancer risk under a dominant genetic model.

Subjects aged <65 years based on 159 cases and 365 controls were genotyped for comparison. There was somewhat difference in the impact of polymorphism on lung cancer risk between subjects aged ≥65 years and those <65 years. Unlike with the results from elderly, *CYP2A6* deletion, *NQO1* rs1800566, and *NAT2* polymor-

Table 11.5 Association between genetic polymorphisms involved in xenobiotic metabolism and lung cancer risk [14, 15, 18, 20, 24, 25]

Polymorphism	Adjusted[a] OR (95% CI)			
	Aged ≥65 years	P	Aged <65 years[b]	P
CYP1A1 rs4646903				
TT	1.0 (reference)		1.0 (reference)	
TC	1.39 (0.84–2.28)	0.196	1.54 (0.94–2.50)	0.084
CC	2.36 (1.13–4.94)	0.022	2.82 (1.47–5.40)	0.002
	$P_{trend} = 0.019$		$P_{trend} = 0.002$	
TC + CC vs. TT	1.58 (0.99–2.53)	0.054	1.80 (1.14–2.85)	0.012
CYP1A1 rs1048943				
Ile/Ile	1.0 (reference)		1.0 (reference)	
Ile/Val	1.62 (0.98–2.68)	0.061	0.89 (0.55–1.44)	0.629
Val/Val	1.73 (0.74–4.01)	0.204	4.09 (1.76–9.53)	0.001
	$P_{trend} = 0.053$		$P_{trend} = 0.033$	
Ile/Val + Val/Val vs. Ile/Ile	1.64 (1.03–2.62)	0.038	1.20 (0.77–1.87)	0.415
CYP1A2 rs762551				
AA	1.0 (reference)		1.0 (reference)	
AC	0.97 (0.58–1.64)	0.936	1.09 (0.68–1.74)	0.730
CC	0.97 (0.47–2.00)	0.935	0.70 (0.34–1.45)	0.336
	$P_{trend} = 0.927$		$P_{trend} = 0.545$	
AC + CC vs. AA	0.98 (0.59–1.61)	0.927	1.00 (0.63–1.57)	0.993
CYP1A2 rs2069514				
AA	0.40 (0.15–1.09)	0.074	0.71 (0.47–1.14)	0.157
AG	0.82 (0.50–1.34)	0.436	1.01 (0.40–2.55)	0.985
GG	1.0 (reference)		1.0 (reference)	
	$P_{trend} = 0.102$		$P_{trend} = 0.358$	
AG + AA vs. GG	0.75 (0.47–1.19)	0.223	0.75 (0.48–1.17)	0.205
CYP2A6 deletion				
*1*1	1.0 (reference)		1.0 (reference)	
*1*4	1.21 (0.69–2.13)	0.498	1.71 (1.01–2.92)	0.049
*4*4 (deletion)	NA		2.87 (0.53–15.5)	0.221
			$P_{trend} = 0.024$	
*1*4 + *4*4 vs. *1*1	1.28 (0.73–2.24)	0.387	1.78 (1.06–2.99)	0.029
CYP2A13 rs8192789				
Arg/Arg	1.0 (reference)		1.0 (reference)	
Arg/Cys	1.26 (0.70–2.29)	0.438	0.98 (0.55–1.76)	0.950
Cys/Cys	3.13 (0.37–26.5)	0.295	2.60 (0.63–10.8)	0.189
	$P_{trend} = 0.220$		$P_{trend} = 0.450$	
Arg/Cys + Cys/Cys vs. Arg/Arg	1.36 (0.76–2.41)	0.297	1.11 (0.64–1.92)	0.708
CYP2E1 rs2031920				
CC	1.0 (reference)		1.0 (reference)	
CT	0.82 (0.51–1.34)	0.435	0.81 (0.50–1.32)	0.406

(continued)

Table 11.5 (continued)

Polymorphism	Adjusted[a] OR (95% CI) Aged ≥65 years	P	Aged <65 years[b]	P
TT	NA		0.69 (0.22–2.14)	0.523
			P_{trend} = 0.325	
CT + TT vs. CC	0.90 (0.56–1.46)	0.679	0.80 (0.50–1.27)	0.341
MPO rs2333227				
AA	NA		0.36 (0.03–3.77)	0.395
GA	0.63 (0.33–1.19)	0.152	1.04 (0.58–1.87)	0.887
GG	1.0 (reference)		1.0 (reference)	
	P_{trend} = 0.285		P_{trend} = 0.771	
GA + AA vs. GG	0.66 (0.36–1.24)	0.201	0.98 (0.56–1.73)	0.949
GSTM1 deletion				
Non-null	1.0 (reference)		1.0 (reference)	
Null	1.61 (1.01–2.55)	0.043	1.23 (0.79–1.91)	0.359
GSTT1 deletion				
Non-null	1.0 (reference)		1.0 (reference)	
Null	1.21 (0.76–1.92)	0.413	1.16 (0.75–1.79)	0.510
GSTP1 rs1695				
Ile/Ile	1.0 (reference)		1.0 (reference)	
Ile/Val	2.18 (1.22–3.89)	0.008	0.92 (0.55–1.53)	0.739
Val/Val	2.94 (0.59–14.7)	0.189	3.70 (0.93–14.6)	0.062
	P_{trend} = 0.005		P_{trend} = 0.429	
Ile/Val + Val/Val vs. Ile/Ile	2.25 (1.29–3.92)	0.004	1.06 (0.65–1.73)	0.827
NQO1 rs1800566				
Pro/Pro	1.0 (reference)		1.0 (reference)	
Pro/Ser	1.12 (0.66–1.91)	0.666	1.51 (0.90–2.55)	0.121
Ser/Ser	1.41 (0.71–2.78)	0.319	2.18 (1.18–4.02)	0.013
	P_{trend} = 0.329		P_{trend} = 0.329	
Pro/Ser + Ser/Ser vs. Pro/Pro	1.20 (0.73–1.97)	0.477	1.70 (1.04–2.78)	0.033
SULT1A1 rs9282861				
Arg/Arg	1.0 (reference)		1.0 (reference)	
Arg/His	1.63 (0.99–2.68)	0.056	1.70 (1.06–2.74)	0.029
His/His	1.99 (0.22–18.1)	0.542	2.44 (0.48–12.4)	0.281
	P_{trend} = 0.052		P_{trend} = 0.018	
Arg/His + His/His vs. Arg/Arg	1.64 (1.001–2.69)	0.050	174 (1.09–2.77)	0.020
NAT2[c]				
Rapid acetylator (RA)	1.0 (reference)		1.0 (reference)	
Intermediate acetylator (IA)	1.59 (0.86–2.94)	0.143	2.09 (1.20–3.62)	0.009
Slow acetylator (SA)	1.19 (0.59–2.40)	0.625	1.69 (0.87–3.27)	0.121
	P_{trend} = 0.775		P_{trend} = 0.104	
IA + SA vs. RA	1.45 (0.80–2.62)	0.217	1.97 (1.16–3.34)	0.012

OR odds ratio, *95% CI* 95% confidence interval, *NA* not available
[a]Adjusted for age, sex, education, smoking status, and drinking status
[b]Based on 159 cases and 265 controls
[c]Genotypes determined by *NAT2*4, *5B, *6A, or *7B allele. Rapid acetylator, *4/*4; intermediate acetylator, *4/*5B, *4/*6A, *4/*7B; slow acetylator, *5B/*5B, *5B/*6A, *5B/*7B, *6A/*6A*6A/*7B, *7B/*7B

phisms were significantly associated with lung cancer risk. *GSTM1* deletion and *GSTP1* rs1695 polymorphisms were not significantly associated with lung cancer risk. As there was an overlap between the CIs of the ORs for each polymorphism in the two groups, it can be assumed that there is no statistically significant difference in the ORs between the two groups.

11.2.3.3 Association Between Genetic Polymorphisms Involved in DNA Repair and Lung Cancer Risk

The genotype frequencies of six polymorphisms were all in agreement with the HWE in controls (data not shown). As shown in Table 11.6 [16, 18, 24], only *TP53BP1* rs560191 was significantly associated with lung cancer risk. The ORs of lung cancer for the Glu/Glu genotype and Asp/Glu genotype were 0.40 (95% CI = 0.20–0.80) and 0.56 (95% CI = 0.33–0.95), respectively. Decreasing numbers of the Asp allele decreased lung cancer risk in a dose-dependent manner (P_{trend} = 0.006). A statistically significant decreased lung cancer risk was found under dominant model (OR = 0.51, 95% CI = 0.31–0.85).

Unlike with the results from elderly, *ERCC2* rs13181 and *XRCC1* rs25487 polymorphisms were significantly associated with lung cancer risk among subjects aged <65 years. As there was an overlap between the CIs of the ORs for each polymorphism, the differences are not statistically significant.

11.2.3.4 Association Between Genetic Polymorphisms Involved in Inflammation and Lung Cancer Risk

The genotype frequencies of 11 polymorphisms were in agreement with the HWE in controls, except for *CYBA* rs4673 in the elderly group (P = 0.039) and *IL1B1* rs1143634 in the non-elderly group (P = 0.028). Table 11.7 illustrates association between genetic polymorphisms involved in inflammation and lung cancer risk [17, 19, 21, 26]. The CT genotype of *CRP* rs2794520 (OR = 1.67, 95% CI = 1.02–2.73) was significantly associated with an increased risk of lung cancer. A statistically significant increased lung cancer risk was found under dominant model (OR = 1.73, 95% CI = 1.09–2.76). A dose-dependent relationship (P_{trend} = 0.024) was revealed between number of the C (T) allele and lung cancer risk. There was little difference in the impact of polymorphism on lung cancer risk between elderly and non-elderly subjects.

11.2.4 *Discussion*

The selected 31 polymorphisms involved in xenobiotic metabolism, DNA repair, and inflammatory response were determined in a total of 417 elderly subjects (303 lung cancer cases and 114 controls) and 424 non-elderly subjects (159 lung cancer

Table 11.6 Association between genetic polymorphisms involved in DNA repair and lung cancer risk [16, 18, 24]

Polymorphism	Adjusted[a] OR (95% CI)			
	Aged ≥65 years	P	Aged <65 years[b]	P
ERCC2 rs13181				
Lys/Lys	1.0 (reference)		1.0 (reference)	
Lys/Gln	0.97 (0.55–1.69)	0.910	2.61 (1.47–4.64)	0.001
Gln/Gln	1.31 (0.25–7.04)	0.750	9.73 (2.84–33.3)	<0.0001
	$P_{trend} = 0.936$		$P_{trend} < 0.0001$	
Lys/Gln + Gln/Gln vs. Lys/Lys	0.99 (0.58–1.70)	0.984	3.26 (1.90–5.58)	<0.0001
XRCC1 rs25487				
Arg/Arg	1.0 (reference)		1.0 (reference)	
Arg/Gln	0.98 (0.60–1.61)	0.952	1.81 (1.12–2.92)	0.016
Gln/Gln	1.74 (0.76–4.00)	0.191	4.20 (1.55–11.4)	0.005
	$P_{trend} = 0.335$		$P_{trend} = 0.001$	
Arg/Gln + Gln/Gln vs. Arg/Arg	1.12 (0.70–1.77)	0.644	2.04 (1.29–3.23)	0.002
XRCC3 rs861539				
Thr/Thr	1.0 (reference)		1.0 (reference)	
Thr/Met	0.82 (0.48–1.38)	0.453	1.10 (0.62–1.92)	0.745
Met/Met	1.05 (0.21–5.33)	0.952	1.59 (0.42–5.94)	0.494
	$P_{trend} = 0.559$		$P_{trend} = 0.510$	
Thr/Met + Met/Met vs. Thr/Thr	0.83 (0.50–1.39)	0.486	1.15 (0.68–1.95)	0.603
OGG1 rs1052133				
Ser/Ser	0.62 (0.32–1.18)	0.146	0.84 (0.49–1.45)	0.538
Cys/Ser	0.75 (0.41–1.37)	0.347	0.89 (0.49–1.62)	0.714
Cys/Cys	1.0 (reference)		1.0 (reference)	
	$P_{trend} = 0.148$		$P_{trend} = 0.723$	
Cys/Ser + Ser/Ser vs. Cys/Cys	0.69 (0.39–1.22)	0.206	0.86 (052–1.42)	0.563
TP53 rs1042522				
Pro/Pro	1.00 (0.17–2.14)	0.991	1.24 (0.61–2.52)	0.547
Pro/Arg	0.72 (0.44–1.17)	0.185	1.01 (0.63–1.60)	0.972
Arg/Arg	1.0 (reference)		1.0 (reference)	
	$P_{trend} = 0.574$		$P_{trend} = 0.635$	
Pro/Arg + Pro/Pro vs. Arg/Arg	0.77 (0.48–1.23)	0.276	1. 05 (0.68–1.64)	0.816
TP53BP1 rs560191				
Asp/Asp	1.0 (reference)		1.0 (reference)	
Asp/Glu	0.56 (0.33–0.95)	0.033	1.14 (0.70–1.87)	0.602
Glu/Glu	0.40 (0.20–0.80)	0.009	0.45 (0.22–0.61)	0.026
	$P_{trend} = 0.006$		$P_{trend} = 0.078$	
Asp/Glu + Glu/Glu vs. Asp/Asp	0.51 (0.31–0.85)	0.009	0.92 (0.58–1.48)	0.737

OR odds ratio, *95% CI* 95% confidence interval
[a]Adjusted for age, sex, education, smoking status, and drinking status
[b]Based on 159 cases and 265 controls

Table 11.7 Association between genetic polymorphisms involved in inflammation and lung cancer risk [17, 19, 21, 26]

Polymorphism	Adjusted[a] OR (95% CI)				
	Aged ≥65 years	P	Aged <65 years[b]	P	
IL1B rs1143634					
CC	1.0 (reference)		1.0 (reference)		
CT	1.15 (0.60–2.21)	0.677	1.48 (0.77–2.86)	0.244	
TT	NA		1.77 (0.28–11.2)	0.543	
			$P_{trend} = 0.201$		
CT + TT vs. CC	1.33 (0.70–2.54)	0.384	1.51 (0.80–2.83)	0.200	
IL6 rs1800796					
CC	1.0 (reference)		1.0 (reference)		
CG	1.53 (0.92–2.53)	0.100	1.21 (0.75–1.95)	0.427	
GG	0.98 (0.37–2.65)	0.976	3.39 (1.13–10.2)	0.029	
	$P_{trend} = 0.281$		$P_{trend} = 0.057$		
CG + GG vs. CC	1.43 (0.89–2.31)	0.141	1.37 (0.87–2.16)	0.174	
IL8 rs4073					
TT	1.0 (reference)		1.0 (reference)		
TA	0.71 (0.44–1.64)	0.176	1.40 (0.88–2.23)	0.158	
AA	1.13 (0.50–2.55)	0.766	0.82 (0.36–1.85)	0.638	
	$P_{trend} = 0.684$		$P_{trend} = 0.668$		
TA + AA vs. TT	0.78 (0.48–1.24)	0.294	1.27 (0.82–1.97)	0.290	
IL10 rs1800871					
CC	0.94 (0.46–1.93)	0.877	1.61 (0.78–3.33)	0.201	
CT	1.15 (0.69–1.91)	0.589	1.45 (0.91–2.31)	0.121	
TT	1.0 (reference)		1.0 (reference)		
	$P_{trend} = 0.942$		$P_{trend} = 0.097$		
CT + CC vs. TT	1.10 (0.68–1.77)	0.699	1.48 (0.95–2.31)	0.086	
IL13 rs1800925					
CC	1.0 (reference)		1.0 (reference)		
CT	0.94 (0.58–1.53)	0.814	1.47 (0.91–2.31)	0.117	
TT	3.32 (0.41–27.0)	0.261	1.15 (0.40–3.27)	0.796	
	$P_{trend} = 0.698$		$P_{trend} = 0.209$		
CT + TT vs. CC	1.01 (0.63–1.62)	0.976	1.42 (0.90–2.34)	0.132	
CRP rs2794520					
CC	2.03 (0.87–4.75)	0.103	1.98 (0.92–4.24)	0.080	
CT	1.67 (1.02–2.73)	0.040	1.58 (0.99–2.52)	0.057	
TT	1.0 (reference)		1.0 (reference)		
	$P_{trend} = 0.024$		$P_{trend} = 0.028$		
CT + CC vs. TT	1.73 (1.09–2.76)	0.021	1.64 (1.05–2.57)	0.031	
NOS2 rs2297518					
CC	1.0 (reference)		1.0 (reference)		
CT	1.02 (0.53–1.96)	0.962	1.32 (0.70–2.51)	0.391	

(continued)

Table 11.7 (continued)

Polymorphism	Adjusted[a] OR (95% CI)			
	Aged ≥65 years	P	Aged <65 years[b]	P
TT	NA		1.80 (0.19–16.9)	0.606
			$P_{trend} = 0.326$	
CT + TT vs. CC	1.04 (0.54–2.00)	0.900	1.35 (0.73–2.51)	0.343
CYBA rs4673				
CC	1.0 (reference)		1.0 (reference)	
CT	1.01 (0.49–2.11)	0.972	1.23 (0.67–2.28)	0.501
TT	0.66 (0.10–4.20)	0.661	5.75 (0.46–72.0)	0.175
	$P_{trend} = 0.821$		$P_{trend} = 0.233$	
CT + TT vs. CC	0.96 (0.48–1.92)	0.917	1.33 (0.73–2.43)	0.348
TNFA rs1799724				
CC	1.0 (reference)		1.0 (reference)	
CT	1.28 (0.76–2.14)	0.355	1.07 (0.66–1.73)	0.798
TT	0.93 (0.30–2.91)	0.903	1.64 (0.50–5.45)	0.416
	$P_{trend} = 0.552$		$P_{trend} = 0.513$	
CT + TT vs. CC	1.23 (0.75–2.00)	0.418	1.11 (0.70–1.77)	0.646
TNFRA2 rs1061622				
GG	1.52 (0.47–4.91)	0.484	0.94 (0.20–4.28)	0.932
TG	1.64 (0.49–5.51)	0.424	0.89 (0.19–4.19)	0.932
TT	1.0 (reference)		1.0 (reference)	
	$P_{trend} = 0.859$		$P_{trend} = 0.887$	
TG + GG vs. TT	1.55 (0.49–4.97)	0.455	0.92 (0.20–4.19)	0.916
NFkB rs28362491				
DD	0.54 (0.26–1.16)	0.114	0.72 (0.36–1.46)	0.366
ID	0.70 (0.43–1.15)	0.160	0.84 (0.53–1.33)	0.452
II	1.0 (reference)		1.0 (reference)	
	$P_{trend} = 0.068$		$P_{trend} = 0.309$	
ID + DD vs. II	0.67 (0.42–1.06)	0.090	0.81 (0.52–1.26)	0.351

OR odds ratio, *95% CI* 95% confidence interval, *NA* not available
[a]Adjusted for age, sex, smoking status, drinking status, and education
[b]Based on 159 cases and 265 controls

patients and 265 controls). Seven polymorphisms, namely, *CYP1A1* rs4646903, *CYP1A1* rs1048943, *GSTM1* deletion, *GSTP1* rs1695, *SULTA1* rs9282861, *TP53BP1* rs560191, and *CRP* rs2794520, were associated with lung cancer risk in the elderly group. *CYP2E1* rs2031920 and *CYBA* rs4673 in elderly controls and *IL1B1* rs1143634 in non-elderly controls deviated from HWE.

In our previous case-control studies [14, 16–19, 21, 27, 28], the minor homozygotes of *CYP1A1* rs4646903 (OR = 2.63, 95% CI = 1.61–4.28), *CYP1A1* rs1048943 (OR = 2.86, 95% CI = 1.54–5.32), *GSTP1* rs1695 (OR = 3.22, 95% CI = 1.12–9.30), *CRP* rs2794520 (OR = 1.92, 95% CI = 1.10–3.38), and *TP53BP1* rs560191 (OR = 0.46, 95% CI = 0.29–0.74) were significantly associated with an increased lung cancer risk in the whole population (462 lung cancer cases and 379 controls).

Similarly, the null genotype of the *GSTM1* deletion polymorphism was at a 1.38-fold (95% CI = 1.01–1.89) increased risk of lung cancer 1.38 (1.01–1.89) in the whole population. Although the authors did not report the association between *SULT1A1* rs9282861 and lung cancer risk, *SULT1A1* rs9282861 was associated with lung cancer risk under dominant model (OR = 1.33, 95% CI = 1.00–1.76, *P* = 0.05) in a recent meta-analysis [29]. The observed ORs of lung cancer for these polymorphisms were consistent with those from a considerable amount of studies, including our previous studies, but attenuated due to a reduced sample size. Basically, the impact of selected genetic polymorphisms on lung cancer may be similar between the elderly population and the non-elderly population. Our findings suggest the impact of selected genetic polymorphisms on lung cancer is independent of age.

Departure from HWE can imply the presence of selection bias (lack of representation of the general population) in this population because this study was free from the possibility of genotyping error (e.g., systematic misgenotyping of heterozygotes as homozygotes or vice versa or nonrandomness of missing data), assay nonspecificity, or possible population admixture/stratification [30, 31]. The Japanese population sample could be expected to have a relatively low risk of population stratification effects [32, 33] in comparison to Caucasian populations that have a geographically broader-based inheritance. The deviation from HWE is most likely due to chance. For example, no controls had the TT genotype of *CYP2E1* rs2031920 in this study. If one control had possessed the TT genotype, there was no longer a deviation from HWE in controls (*P* = 0.053). On the other hand, two controls had the TT genotype of *CYBA* rs4673. If one control had possessed the TT genotype, there was no longer a deviation from HWE in controls (*P* = 0.359). It is plausible that the deviation from HWE was due to chance in this study.

Understanding the genetic basis of complex diseases has been increasingly emphasized as a means of achieving insight into disease pathogenesis, with the ultimate goal of improving preventive strategies, diagnostic tools, and therapies. Case-control genetic association studies such as ours aim to detect association between genetic polymorphisms and disease. Although case-control genetic association studies can measure statistical associations, they cannot test causality. Determining genetic causation of disease is a process of inference, which requires supportive results from multiple association studies and basic science experiments combined. Furthermore, a concern with respect to genetic association studies has been lack of replication studies, especially contradictory findings across studies. Replication of findings is very important before any causal inference can be drawn. Testing replication in different populations is an important step. Additional studies are warranted to replicate our and others' findings from case-control genetic association studies.

In summary, *CYP1A1* rs4646903, *CYP1A1* rs1048943, *GSTM1* deletion, *GSTP1* rs1695, *SULTA1* rs9282861, *TP53BP1* rs560191, and *CRP* rs2794520 were associated with lung cancer risk in the elderly population. The impact of selected genetic polymorphisms on lung cancer is independent of age. Future studies involving larger control and case populations will undoubtedly lead to a more thorough understanding of the role of genetic polymorphisms in lung cancer development among elderly.

11.3   Conclusion

Our health status in the later life is influenced by the life experience throughout life. Therefore, health promotion to reduce the risk of chronic diseases such as cancers is important to obtain healthy aging. Lung cancer is the most common cancer worldwide [34], which is the leading cause of cancer death in Japan [1].

Similar to the population as a whole, to adequately control risk factors for lung cancer, such as avoiding the exposure of harmful cigarette smoke and increasing fruits consumption [4–6] (Table 11.3), might be linked to a healthy life and/or a longer life expectancy of the elderly. For example, even a 60-year-old cigarette smoker could gain at least 3 years of life expectancy by stopping [35]. It is accepted that oxidative damage contributes greatly to the aging process and the development of various diseases [36]. Antioxidants can decrease the oxidative damage by reacting with free radicals or by inhibiting their activity. Fruits are a source of vitamin C and other antioxidants such as carotenoids, flavonoids, and polyphenols. Therefore, fruits can be used to benefit human health issues related to retarding aging (increase in life expectancy). Due to prolonging life expectancy and the increased risk of lung cancer with aging, lung cancer is common in the elderly. As lung cancer has a relatively long latency period from the time of initial exposure to the onset of symptoms, anti-smoking education programs should be introduced at an early age.

In addition to primary prevention, secondary prevention (i.e., early detection of asymptomatic lung cancer) is also important for our good health status in the later life. Among both men and women, the incidence of lung cancer is low in persons under age 45 and increases with age [4]. Therefore, screening for lung cancer after the middle ages is important to detect asymptomatic lung cancer as well as to avoid unhealthy aging.

Krabbe and Lotan suggested to us that newly diagnosed bladder cancer patients should also be screened for lung cancer because a small number (i.e., 4–5%) of bladder cancer patients were also diagnosed with lung cancer [37]. As bladder cancer and lung cancer have shared risk factors (i.e., tobacco smoking [8] and arsenic in drinking water [38]) and inherited susceptibility (i.e., GSM1 deletion polymorphism and NAT2 [39]) and lung cancer is the most common death from cancer, it is appropriate that Krabbe and Lotan recommend urologists to advise bladder cancer patients to undergo screening of lung cancer [40]. Therefore, we should advise patients with smoking-related cancers other than lung cancer to undergo screening for lung cancer because tobacco smoking is associated with an increased risk of malignancies of both organs in direct contact with smoke and organs not in direct contact with smoke [3].

In addition to environmental factors, a substantial number of genetic polymorphisms have been determined as possible risk factors for lung cancer [41–43]. Global estimates suggest that approximately 25% of lung cancer cases worldwide occur among never smokers [44, 45]. Family history has been reported a simple proxy for genetic risk and is influenced by both shared and individual environmental exposures [46]. Understanding the underlying genetic factors will have a high degree of availability for clarifying the etiology of lung cancer and in identifying high-risk individuals for targeted screening and/or prevention based on a combination of genetic and environmental factors in the elderly population as well as the population as a whole.

In the end, the impact of genetic factors on lung cancer may be unrelated to age. Tobacco smoking is the best established and strongest avoidable risk factor for lung cancer. Although tobacco smoking is associated with an increased risk of malignancies of both organs in direct contact with smoke and organs not in direct contact with smoke [3] as well as an increased risk of cardiovascular diseases or chronic obstructive pulmonary disease [47], more than 30% of Japanese boys experienced tobacco smoking before becoming junior high school students [48, 49], and more than 10% of Japanese girls did so before becoming senior high school students [49]. As healthy aging is a lifelong process, anti-smoking education from an early age and the prevention of tobacco smoking throughout the lifetime are important for healthy aging.

References

1. Health, Labour and Welfare Statistics Association. Trend of national health 2017/2018. Tokyo: Health, Labour and Welfare Statistics Association; 2017 (in Japanese).
2. Thun MJ, Henley SJ. Tobacco. In: Schottenfeld D, Fraumeni Jr JF, editors. Cancer epidemiology and prevention. New York: Oxford University Press; 1996. p. 217–42.
3. Gajalakshmi CK, Jha P, Ranson K, Nguyen S. Global patterns of smoking and smoking-attributable mortality. In: Jha P, Chalouplca F, editors. Tobacco control in developing countries. New York: Oxford University Press; 2000. p. 11–39.
4. Boffetta P, Trichopoulos D. Cancer of the lung, larynx, and pleura. In: Adami HO, Hunter D, Trichopoulos D, editors. Text of cancer epidemiology. New York: Oxford University Press; 2002. p. 248–80.
5. World Cancer Research Fund/American Institute for Cancer Research. Food, nutrition, physical activity, and the prevention of cancer: a global perspective. Washington, DC: AICR/WCRF; 2007.
6. http://epi.ncc.go.jp/files/02_can_prev/matrix_170801JP.pdf (ver. 20170801).
7. Washio M, Tanaka Y, Inomata S, Takahashi H, Saitoh S, Miura T, et al. Smoking increases the risk of lung cancer while green tea and green and yellow vegetables reduces the risk: a case-control study of lung cancer in Hokkaido. Rinsho To Kenkyu. 2016;93(1):93–6 (in Japanese).
8. Doll R, Peto R. The causes of cancer: quantitative estimates of avoidable risks of cancer in the United States today. J Natl Cancer Inst. 1981;66(6):1191–308.
9. Tafani M, Sansone L, Limana F, Arcangeli T, De Santis E, Polese M, et al. The interplay of reactive oxygen species, hypoxia, inflammation, and sirtuins in cancer initiation and progression. Oxidative Med Cell Longev. 2016;2016:3907147. https://doi.org/10.1155/2016/3907147.
10. Nebert DW. Role of genetics and drug metabolism in human cancer risk. Mutat Res. 1991;247(2):267–81.
11. Bartsch H, Nair J. Chronic inflammation and oxidative stress in the genesis and perpetuation of cancer: role of lipid peroxidation, DNA damage, and repair. Langenbeck's Arch Surg. 2006;391(5):499–510. https://doi.org/10.1007/s00423-006-0073-1.
12. Smith CJ, Perfetti TA, King JA. Perspectives on pulmonary inflammation and lung cancer risk in cigarette smokers. Inhal Toxicol. 2006;18(9):667–77. https://doi.org/10.1080/08958370600742821.

13. Barrera G. Oxidative stress and lipid peroxidation products in cancer progression and therapy. ISRN Oncol. 2012;2012:137289. https://doi.org/10.5402/2012/137289.
14. Kiyohara C, Yamamura KI, Nakanishi Y, Takayama K, Hara N. Polymorphism in GSTM1, GSTT1, and GSTP1 and susceptibility to lung cancer in a Japanese population. Asian Pac J Cancer Prev. 2000;1(4):293–8.
15. Kiyohara C, Takayama K, Nakanishi Y. CYP2A13, CYP2A6, and the risk of lung adenocarcinoma in a Japanese population. J Health Sci. 2005;51(6):658–66. https://doi.org/10.1248/jhs.51.658.
16. Kiyohara C, Horiuchi T, Miyake Y, Takayama K, Nakanishi Y. Cigarette smoking, TP53 Arg72Pro, TP53BP1 Asp353Glu and the risk of lung cancer in a Japanese population. Oncol Rep. 2010;23(5):1361–8.
17. Kiyohara C, Horiuchi T, Takayama K, Nakanishi Y. IL1B rs1143634 polymorphism, cigarette smoking, alcohol use, and lung cancer risk in a Japanese population. J Thorac Oncol. 2010;5(3):299–304. https://doi.org/10.1097/JTO.0b013e3181c8cae3.
18. Kiyohara C, Horiuchi T, Takayama K, Nakanishi Y. Genetic polymorphisms involved in carcinogen metabolism and DNA repair and lung cancer risk in a Japanese population. J Thorac Oncol. 2012;7(6):954–62. https://doi.org/10.1097/JTO.0b013e31824de30f.
19. Kiyohara C, Horiuchi T, Takayama K, Nakanishi Y. Genetic polymorphisms involved in the inflammatory response and lung cancer risk: a case-control study in Japan. Cytokine. 2014;65(1):88–94. https://doi.org/10.1016/j.cyto.2013.09.015.
20. Kakino K, Kiyohara C, Horiuchi T, Nakanishi Y. CYP2E1 rs2031920, COMT rs4680 polymorphisms, cigarette smoking, alcohol use and lung cancer risk in a Japanese population. Asian Pac J Cancer Prev. 2016;17(8):4063–70.
21. Yamamoto Y, Kiyohara C, Suetsugu-Ogata S, Hamada N, Nakanishi Y. Biological interaction of cigarette smoking on the association between genetic polymorphisms involved in inflammation and the risk of lung cancer: a case-control study in Japan. Oncol Lett. 2017;13(5):3873–81. https://doi.org/10.3892/ol.2017.5867.
22. Holman CD, English DR, Milne E, Winter MG. Meta-analysis of alcohol and all-cause mortality: a validation of NHMRC recommendations. Med J Aust. 1996;164(3):141–5.
23. Benedetti A, Parent ME, Siemiatycki J. Lifetime consumption of alcoholic beverages and risk of 13 types of cancer in men: results from a case-control study in Montreal. Cancer Detect Prev. 2009;32(5–6):352–62.
24. Kiyohara C, Nakanishi Y, Takayama K, Horiuchi T, Miyake Y. Molecular epidemiologic study of lung cancer on interaction between smoking and genetic factors. The 2009 Grant-in-Aid for Scientific Research (B) Report (Grant Number: 7390175), Japan Society for the Promotion of Science [cited 1 Feb 2018]. https://kaken.nii.ac.jp/file/KAKENHI-PROJECT-17390175/17390175seika.pdf (in Japanese).
25. Kiyohara C, Nakanishi Y, Horiuchi T, Takayama K. Genome epidemiologic study on lung cancer and estrogen-related genes. The 2017 Grant-in-Aid for Scientific Research (B) Report (Grant Number: 25293143), Japan Society for the Promotion of Science [cited 1 Feb 2018]. https://kaken.nii.ac.jp/file/KAKENHI-PROJECT-25293143/25293143seika.pdf (in Japanese).
26. Kiyohara C, Nakanishi Y, Takayama K, Horiuchi T. Genome epidemiologic study on lung cancer and inflammation-related genes. The 2013 Grant-in-Aid for Scientific Research (B) Report (Grant Number: 21390190), Japan Society for the Promotion of Science [cited 1 Feb 2018]. https://kaken.nii.ac.jp/file/KAKENHI-PROJECT-21390190/21390190seika.pdf (in Japanese).
27. Kiyohara C, Nakanishi Y, Inutsuka S, Takayama K, Hara N, Motohiro A, et al. The relationship between CYP1A1 aryl hydrocarbon hydroxylase activity and lung cancer in a Japanese population. Pharmacogenetics. 1998;8(4):315–23.
28. Kiyohara C, Horiuchi T, Takayama K, Nakanishi Y. Methylenetetrahydrofolate reductase polymorphisms and interaction with smoking and alcohol consumption in lung cancer

risk: a case-control study in a Japanese population. BMC Cancer. 2011;11:459. https://doi. org/10.1186/1471-2407-11-459.

29. Liao SG, Liu L, Zhang YY, Wang Y, Wang YJ. SULT1A1 Arg213His polymorphism and lung cancer risk: a meta-analysis. Asian Pac J Cancer Prev. 2012;13(2):579–83.

30. Hosking L, Lumsden S, Lewis K, Yeo A, McCarthy L, Bansal A, et al. Detection of genotyping errors by hardy-Weinberg equilibrium testing. Eur J Hum Genet. 2004;12(5):395–9. https:// doi.org/10.1038/sj.ejhg.5201164.

31. Gomes I, Collins A, Lonjou C, Thomas NS, Wilkinson J, Watson M, et al. Hardy-Weinberg quality control. Ann Hum Genet. 1999;63(Pt 6):535–8. https://doi.org/10.1017/S0003480099007824.

32. Haga H, Yamada R, Ohnishi Y, Nakamura Y, Tanaka T. Gene-based SNP discovery as part of the Japanese Millennium Genome Project: identification of 190,562 genetic variations in the human genome. Single-nucleotide polymorphism. J Hum Genet. 2002;47(11):605–10. https:// doi.org/10.1007/s100380200092.

33. Yamaguchi-Kabata Y, Nakazono K, Takahashi A, Saito S, Hosono N, Kubo M, et al. Japanese population structure, based on SNP genotypes from 7003 individuals compared to other ethnic groups: effects on population-based association studies. Am J Hum Genet. 2008;83(4):445–56. https://doi.org/10.1016/j.ajhg.2008.08.019.

34. WHO. Lung cancer. In: Stewart BW, Kleihues P, editors. World cancer report. Lyon: International Agency for Research on Cancer Press; 2003. p. 182–7.

35. Doll R, Peto R, Boreham J, Sutherland I. Mortality in relation to smoking: 50 years' observations on male British doctors. BMJ. 2004;328(7455):1519. https://doi.org/10.1136/bmj.38142.554479.AE.

36. Riscuta G. Nutrigenomics at the interface of aging, lifespan, and cancer prevention. J Nutr. 2016;146(10):1931–9. https://doi.org/10.3945/jn.116.235119.

37. Krabbe LM, Lotan Y. Should patients newly diagnosed with bladder cancer be screened for lung cancer? Int J Urol. 2016;23(4):346–7. https://doi.org/10.1111/iju.13052.

38. International Agency for Research on Cancer. Some drinking-water disinfectants and contaminants, including arsenic, vol. 84. Lyon: World Health Organization; 2004.

39. Hietanen E, Husgafvel-Pursiainen K, Vainio H. Interaction between dose and susceptibility to environmental cancer: a short review. Environ Health Perspect. 1997;105(Suppl 4):749–54.

40. Washio M. Editorial comment to should patients newly diagnosed with bladder cancer be screened for lung cancer? Int J Urol. 2016;23(4):347. https://doi.org/10.1111/iju.13064.

41. Truong T, Sauter W, McKay JD, Hosgood HD 3rd, Gallagher C, Amos CI, et al. International Lung Cancer Consortium: coordinated association study of 10 potential lung cancer susceptibility variants. Carcinogenesis. 2010;31(4):625–33. https://doi.org/10.1093/carcin/bgq001.

42. Hung RJ, Christiani DC, Risch A, Popanda O, Haugen A, Zienolddiny S, et al. International Lung Cancer Consortium: pooled analysis of sequence variants in DNA repair and cell cycle pathways. Cancer Epidemiol Biomarkers Prev. 2008;17(11):3081–9. https://doi.org/10.1158/1055-9965.Epi-08-0411.

43. Kiyohara C, Yoshimasu K, Takayama K, Nakanishi Y. Lung cancer susceptibility: are we on our way to identifying a high-risk group? Future Oncol (London, England). 2007;3(6):617–27. https://doi.org/10.2217/14796694.3.6.617.

44. Parkin DM, Bray F, Ferlay J, Pisani P. Global cancer statistics, 2002. CA Cancer J Clin. 2005;55(2):74–108.

45. Sun S, Schiller JH, Gazdar AF. Lung cancer in never smokers—a different disease. Nat Rev Cancer. 2007;7(10):778–90. https://doi.org/10.1038/nrc2190.

46. Cote ML, Liu M, Bonassi S, Neri M, Schwartz AG, Christiani DC, et al. Increased risk of lung cancer in individuals with a family history of the disease: a pooled analysis from the International Lung Cancer Consortium. Eur J Cancer. 2012;48(13):1957–68. https://doi.org/10.1016/j.ejca.2012.01.038.

47. Jamrozik K. Tobacco and cardiovascular disease. In: Boyle P, Gray N, Henningfield J, Seffrin J, Zatonski W, editors. Tobacco and public health: science and policy. New York: Oxford University Press Inc.; 2004. p. 549–76. ISBN: 0-19-852687-3.
48. Washio M, Kiyohara C, Morioka S, Mori M. The experiences of smoking in school children up to and including high school ages and the current status of smoking habits; a survey of male high school students in Japan. Asian Pac J Cancer Prev. 2003;4:344–51.
49. Washio M, Kiyohara C, Oura A, Mori M. Smoking in youth: a review. In: Lapointe MM, editor. Adolescent smoking and health research. New York: Nova Science Publishers Inc.; 2008. p. 191–205. ISBN: 987-1-60456-046-6.

Chapter 12
Influenza and Influenza Vaccination in Japanese Elderly

Megumi Hara

Abstract Seasonal influenza epidemics occur every winter. In Japan, this season begins from late November to early December and ends in April to May. According to the National Epidemiological Surveillance of Infectious Disease, around 15 million people, which is about 10% of the entire Japanese population, is estimated to be infected every season. Elderly people account for about 10% of all reported patients; however, their cases may become severe and lead to complications such as pneumonia or result in death. As a countermeasure against influenza in elderly people, an inactivated tetravalent vaccine has been recommended as part of the national immunization program since 2017 in Japan.

This chapter describes the characteristics of influenza virus, influenza disease burden in elderly people, and influenza vaccine as an influenza countermeasure and its effectiveness.

Keywords Influenza virus · Influenza vaccine · Effectiveness · Immunogenicity · Epidemiology

12.1 Influenza Virus

Influenza virus is an RNA virus belonging to the family Orthomyxoviridae, and it is classified into types A, B, and C according to the antigenicity of internal proteins. Epidemic disease in human is caused by influenza A and B viruses. These types are further subclassified based on differences in antigenicity. Influenza A virus is subclassified into subtypes by two surface antigens, hemagglutinin (HA) and neuraminidase (NA). HA, which has 18 subtypes, is necessary for viral attachment to cell surfaces and involved in infection and protection. NA, which has 11 subtypes, acts when the virus proliferates in the cell and escapes out of the cell. Influenza B

M. Hara
Faculty of Medicine, Department of Preventive Medicine, Saga University,
Saga City, Saga, Japan
e-mail: harameg@cc.saga-u.ac.jp

© Springer Nature Singapore Pte Ltd. 2019
M. Washio, C. Kiyohara (eds.), *Health Issues and Care System for the Elderly*,
Current Topics in Environmental Health and Preventive Medicine,
https://doi.org/10.1007/978-981-13-1762-0_12

viruses are classified into two distinct lineages, Yamagata and Victoria, according to genotype, but are not classified as subtypes. Currently, influenza A (H1N1) virus, influenza A (H3N2) virus, and influenza B virus are prevalent in humans. Because influenza virus RNA is divided into eight segments, if influenza viruses of different subtypes infect one cell, genetic reassembly will occur within that cell and mutations within the gene that codes for antigen will occur (antigenic drift). Such minor antigenic drift occurs continuously within both influenza A and B viruses, although influenza B viruses evolve at a slower rate than influenza A viruses. This antigenic drift results in new strains, which cause seasonal epidemics. For this reason, recommended vaccine strains are selected annually.

Influenza A virus infects not only human but also various animals such as birds, pigs, and horses. Therefore, when a gene derived from a human virus and a gene derived from an animal virus are reassembled, a discontinuous mutation (antigenic shift) occurs, resulting in new subtype influenza A viruses that contain a greatly different HA or NA from the virus prevalent until then. Antigenic shift occurs only within influenza A viruses and can lead to a pandemic if the new strain can infect humans and be transmitted from person to person due to little or no preexisting immunity.

Virus type and subtype affect the number of influenza-related deaths and hospitalizations. It is said that influenza A (H3N2) virus epidemic season results in about 2.7 times higher influenza mortality than other types and subtypes compared with the main epidemic season.

12.2 History of Influenza

The history of influenza is considered to have begun in 400 BC, about 2000 years ago. The influenza virus causes annual epidemics of disease and has caused five global pandemics in the last 100 years, resulting in numerous deaths. The estimated number of deaths due to the 1918 Spanish flu pandemic (H1N1 subtype) was about 50 million worldwide, with about 500,000 deaths in Japan. In the 1957 Asian flu pandemic (H3N2 subtype) and 1968 Hong Kong flu pandemic (H3N2 subtype), approximately 3 million people worldwide and 10 million people were affected, respectively [1].

Influenza can spread rapidly in a globalized modern society. In April 2009, the 2009 pandemic influenza A (H1N1) virus was confirmed in Mexico and the United States (USA) and subsequently spread worldwide within a month. The World Health Organization (WHO) declared the disease a pandemic in June. In Japan, affected individuals were confirmed in May, and the pandemic peaked from October to November. This virus was antigenically different from the A(H1N1) virus that had been prevalent in humans from 1977 to 2009, which evolved from a bird-derived influenza A(H1N1) virus that caused the 1918 pandemic. This virus is considered to have invaded both human and pig simultaneously and occurred by gene reassembly. Therefore, during the 2009 pandemic, elderly people born before 1915 were

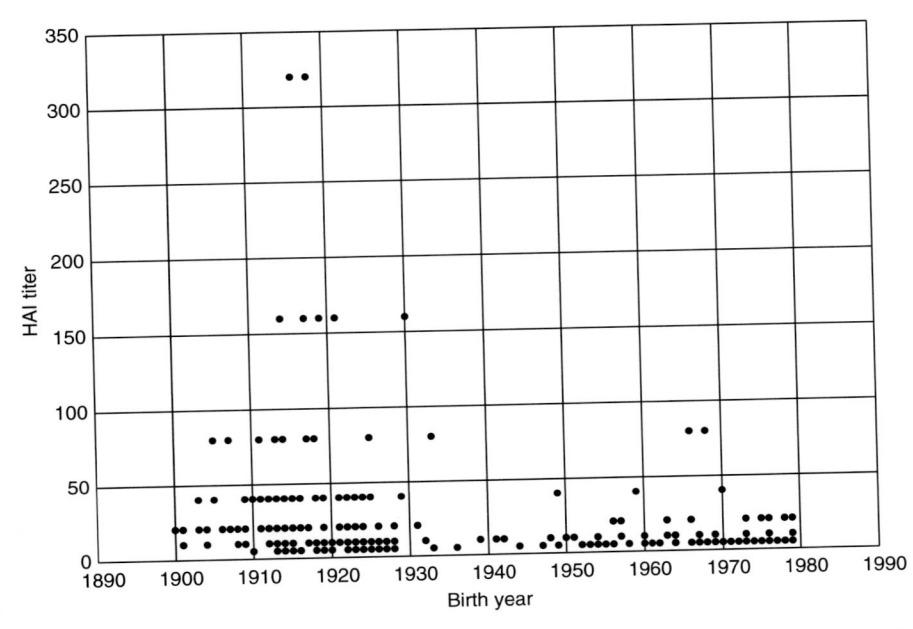

Fig. 12.1 Hemagglutination inhibition (HAI) antibody titers to A(H1N1)pdm09 in serum collected in 2002

reported to have existing antibodies against this virus [2] and cross-reactive neutralizing antibodies against A(H1N1)pdm09 vaccine [3, 4]. The number of deaths from influenza generally increases in older people during the seasonal influenza season; however, the opposite was true during the 2009 pandemic influenza A (H1N1).

The author measured the hemagglutination inhibition (HAI) antibody titer against A(H1N1)pdm09 in 312 stored frozen sera, which were collected from elderly people who were living in nursing homes and institutional staff in 2002. Elderly people born around 1918 had higher HAI antibody titers (Fig. 12.1). Moreover, the proportions of subjects who had antibody against A(H1N1)pdm09 and whose antibody against A(H1N1)pdm09 was ≥1:10 were higher among elderly people born before 1930 (Fig. 12.2).

12.3   Influenza Disease Burden in the Elderly

Influenza is spread from person to person by respiratory tract droplets created by coughing or sneezing. During community outbreaks of seasonal influenza, the highest incidence occurs among children, who account for about 30% of reported cases. However, the numbers of influenza-related hospitalization and deaths are high in the elderly [5]. The proportion of death from influenza-related causes was estimated at 71–85% in the USA [6]. In Japan, hospitalization due to influenza-related disease in

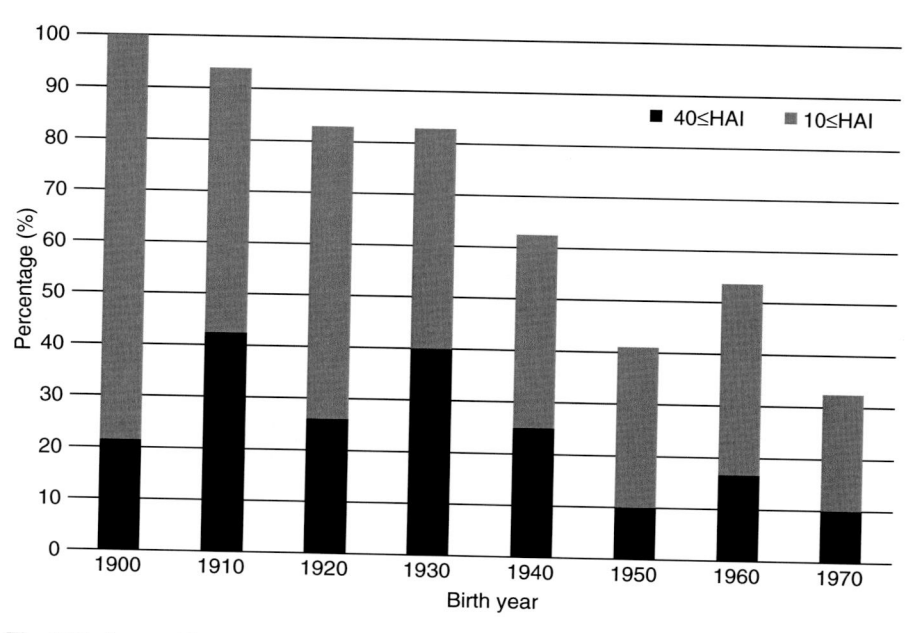

Fig. 12.2 Seropositive proportion against A(H1N1)pdm09 in serum collected in 2002

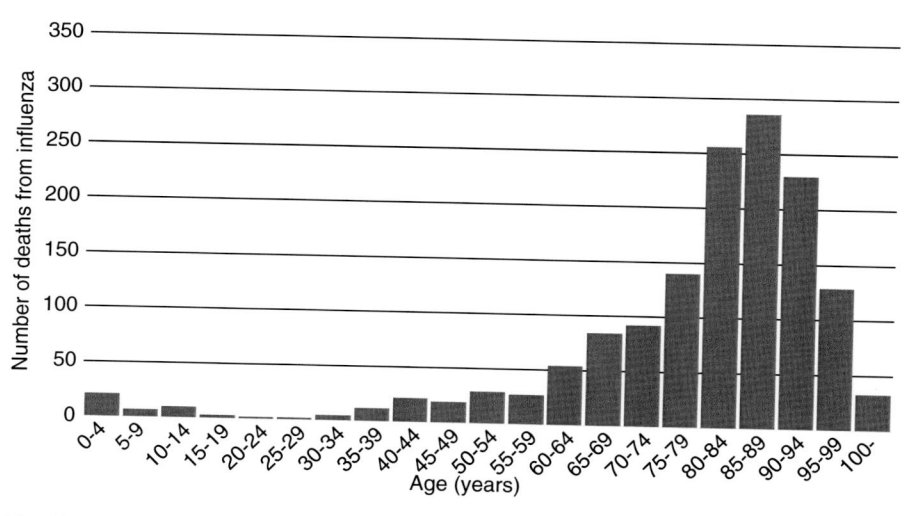

Fig. 12.3 Number of deaths from influenza in Japan, 2016

influenza season is increased with age, and elderly persons (>70 years) accounted for most cases (Fig. 12.3) [5].

One reason for this high rate in elderly persons is that they often live together in nursing homes. Thus, there are many opportunities for person-to-person contact, and influenza infections brought in by healthcare staff and visitors are likely to spread within the facility. In addition, because elderly residents often have underlying diseases and complications and weakened immune systems, influenza infection tends to be serious, often developing into secondary bacterial pneumonia. Therefore, influenza is one of the leading causes of death among the elderly in nursing homes.

12.4   Clinical Symptoms and Treatment of Influenza

Concerning clinical symptoms of influenza in humans, influenza type A generally tends to be more severe than type B. The incubation period of influenza is as short as 1–3 days from infection and characterized by sudden onset. Clinical symptoms of influenza include fever >38 °C, chills, headache, sore throat, nasal obstruction/discharge, cough, muscle pain, joint pain, and general malaise. However, elderly people are less likely to develop high-grade fever because of deteriorated immune defense function, and they may not show typical influenza symptoms. Therefore, during the influenza epidemic period, influenza should be suspected in elderly people who exhibit general fatigue or cough, even if they have a fever <38 °C. In addition, bacterial pneumonia and mixed pneumonia are particularly problematic in the elderly as a complication of seasonal influenza. The frequency of pneumonia complications is especially high when influenza A(H3N2) virus is epidemic. *Streptococcus pneumoniae*, *Haemophilus influenzae*, and *Staphylococcus aureus* are frequently detected as causative bacteria [7].

Supportive care was the major treatment for seasonal influenza until the late 1990s; however, it took 1–2 weeks for symptoms to disappear. In the 2000s, an anti-NA inhibitor was introduced, and antiviral therapy replaced supportive care as the main treatment strategy, subsequently shortening symptom duration and reducing complications. However, serious illness due to pneumonia complications and death remain a problem in the elderly, and disease prevention with vaccines is considered to be important.

12.5   Influenza Vaccine

Influenza virus was discovered in 1933, and vaccine research, development, and improvement have occurred since the 1940s. In Japan, the influenza vaccine was first introduced in 1953. After the 1957 Asian flu pandemic, a special program promoting influenza vaccination among school children was undertaken in 1962. In 1976, the Preventive Vaccination Law was amended to include influenza among the target diseases, and mass vaccination of schoolchildren was started [8]. Sixteen million vaccines were given annually, and the vaccination rate of schoolchildren exceeded 80% until the first half of the 1980s. However, when skepticism about the effectiveness of influenza vaccine appeared in the latter half of the 1980s, vaccination uptake sharply declined. As a result, influenza prevention by vaccine is not anticipated in Japan. Moreover, due to improvements in public health and living standards, the society's concept of vaccination has changed from social defense to inoculation for disease prevention of individuals. Thus, influenza was excluded from the national immunization program according to the Preventive Vaccination Law in 1994. Influenza vaccination became a personal decision, and its uptake drastically decreased. Subsequently, influenza outbreaks occurred in nursing homes, and an increase in influenza-related deaths became a social problem. In 2001, the Preventive Vaccination Law was amended to include influenza vaccination for the elderly in a national immunization program. Recent evaluations speculated that the mass vaccination program for children in the 1970s had indirect effects on influenza-related death of elderly people by suppressing epidemics in the community and transmission to the elderly [9].

Meanwhile, in the USA, influenza has annually been listed as one of the most important diseases for public health measures because it has a fatal influence on elderly people and chronically ill patients. Elderly people and patients with chronic diseases are considered high-risk individuals for influenza, and influenza vaccination has been strongly recommended with the aim of preventing serious complications and deaths in these high-risk individuals. In 1993, the cost of influenza vaccination for the elderly was borne by Medicare (medical insurance for the elderly and physically handicapped), and the vaccination rate increased dramatically. Furthermore, in the 2000s, in order to prevent the spread of influenza to high-risk individuals, the targets of vaccination were expanded to healthcare workers and cohabitants of high-risk people. In 2010, the US vaccination advisory committee recommended influenza vaccination to all individuals older than 6 months [10].

At present, the only available influenza vaccine in Japan is the inactivated tetravalent split vaccine. Virus strains included in the 2017/18 season are A/Singapore/GP1908/2015 (IVR-180) (H1N1)pdm09, A/Hong Kong/4801/2014 (X-263), B/Phuket/3073/2013 (Yamagata lineage), and B/Texas/2/2013 (Victoria lineage). Regarding A(H1N1), the vaccine strain has not changed since the 2009 pandemic. The WHO decides the recommended vaccine strain every February. In Japan, the vaccine strain is determined with reference to the epidemic strain, proliferation, antigenicity, and serum influenza-specific antibody status from the previous season.

The overall influenza vaccination coverage in the influenza season from 2000/2001 to 2010/2011 in Japan was <40% and the vaccination rate for children and elderly people was around 50% [11].

12.5.1 Influenza Vaccine Efficacy and Effectiveness

Vaccine efficacy is derived from the results of a study conducted in an ideal environment, such as randomized clinical trials (RCTs), where the subjects of research are always under the supervision of researchers and the onset situation can be grasped in detail. Vaccine effectiveness is used to describe the results of vaccines in the general population. Vaccine efficacy and effectiveness indicate the percent reduction in the incidence of disease in vaccinated subjects (I_{vac}) compared with the incidence of disease in unvaccinated subjects (I_{unv}) [12] calculated as follows: vaccine efficacy and/or effectiveness = $\{(I_{unv} - I_{vac})/I_{unv}\} \times 100 = \{1 - (I_{vac}/I_{unv})\} \times 100 = \{1 - \text{risk ratio (RR)}\} \times 100$.

Influenza vaccine effectiveness in elderly people is generally considered to be inferior to that in healthy adults. In the 1980s, many retrospective cohort studies in Western countries were conducted by record linkage studies, using large existing administrative datasets, such as those of health maintenance organizations, Medicare, Medicaid, national health insurance schemes, general practice research databases, population and mortality registries, and a vaccination registry database [13]. According to these studies, vaccine effectiveness against influenza of healthy adults was reported as 70–90%, whereas vaccine effectiveness against influenza-related hospitalization of elderly persons living in the community was reported to be 30–70%. Furthermore, concerning elderly persons living in nursing homes, vaccine effectiveness against influenza was reported to be 30–40%, and vaccine effectiveness against influenza-related death was reported to be 80% [13]. However, various biases have been noted in these retrospective studies using large databases. For example, influenza vaccination may be avoided in elderly people who are too frail, but these frail elderly people are likely to develop severe complications if they have influenza. As a result of such bias, vaccine effectiveness will be overestimated if a large number of high-risk individuals are included among unvaccinated individuals. Furthermore, influenza-related pneumonia and hospitalization of elderly people living in the community are recorded in the medical database; thus vaccine effectiveness against these outcome measures can be evaluated. In contrast, vaccine effectiveness against the onset of influenza is not easy to evaluate because such outcomes are not recorded if patients do not visit medical institutions. Therefore, studies such as prospective cohort studies and case-control studies have been conducted.

12.5.2   Influenza Vaccine Effectiveness in Japanese Elderly

In Japan, it is difficult to evaluate influenza vaccine effectiveness using a retrospective cohort study with database linkage because there is no vaccination registration and available database. Therefore, the effectiveness of influenza vaccine against influenza-like illness among community-living elderly people was evaluated by a prospective cohort study [14]. A prospective cohort study to evaluate vaccine effectiveness must observe the target outcome in both vaccinated and unvaccinated subjects over time with "equal intensity." An objective outcome such as "laboratory-confirmed influenza" is the most persuasive evidence of vaccine effectiveness because it reduces the risk of misclassification of outcome for infection. However, in order to use laboratory-confirmed influenza as an outcome, we need to collect information regarding the onset of all influenza-like symptoms from both vaccinated and unvaccinated subjects with equal intensity by frequent contact, such as weekly telephone interviews, then collect respiratory specimens from every participant within a few days, and finally identify influenza virus infection. Thus, such research studies are labor-intensive and costly. Some studies may evaluate vaccine efficacy at the stage of development, but it is difficult to conduct such research on approved vaccines. However, if we use medically confirmed influenza as an outcome, then accurate results cannot be obtained because the likelihood of visits to medical institutions when patients present symptoms depends not only on symptom severity but also on patient characteristics, such as health-conscious behavior. Conversely, laboratory-confirmed influenza may induce ascertainment bias in population-based cohort studies. Vaccinated subjects might not visit medical institutions when they have influenza-related symptoms as compared with unvaccinated subjects because their symptoms might be mild. In contrast, unvaccinated subjects might visit medical institutions more frequently when they have influenza-related symptoms as compared with vaccinated subjects because they might worry about influenza. Thus, unvaccinated subjects tend to be diagnosed as having laboratory-confirmed influenza by passive surveillance in clinical settings, resulting in overestimation of vaccine effectiveness. To avoid such bias, an outcome that can be collected from both vaccinated and unvaccinated subjects with an "equal intensity" must be used.

Therefore, in the prospective cohort study [11], the outcome measure used was influenza-like illness, which was defined as an acute febrile illness with fever >37.8 °C that occurred during the influenza epidemic in the surveyed area, accompanied by symptoms such as nasal discharge, sore throat, cough, and joint pain. We asked study participants to complete a self-reported diary, which included a checklist of symptoms (e.g., cough, sore throat, nasal congestion, muscle ache, and arthralgia), hospital visit, and medication. Active surveillance through monthly telephone interviews by nurses was conducted to ascertain outcomes with equal intensity throughout the influenza season. The study participants or their family members reported their outcomes with reference to the diary records.

In addition, if factors related to both vaccination and outcome measures are "biased" between the vaccinated group and the unvaccinated group, such as the "frail bias" described above, then results are affected. Moreover, elderly people who have chronic disease tend to be vaccinated because they are regularly advised at medical institutions and recommended to be vaccinated. At the same time, elderly people with influenza are likely to develop severe disease because they have underlying disease. As a result, a large number of high-risk individuals are included in the vaccinated group, and then the vaccine effectiveness is difficult to be detected due to such confounding. Potential confounders must be collected at survey baseline and adjusted for during statistical analysis. In this study, we asked subjects about possible confounders, such as age, sex, race, socioeconomic status, residence, comorbid conditions, daycare use, health-conscious behavior, and vaccination history of influenza, using a self-administered questionnaire at the beginning of the study. These factors may be independently related to both risk of influenza and vaccination status; therefore, we adjusted them by multivariate analysis. The occurrence of influenza-like illness during the study period was 24/1000 people. The vaccine effectiveness against influenza-like illness with fever >38.5 °C was estimated to be 62% [95% confidence interval (CI): 15–83%] [14].

12.5.3 Influenza Vaccine Effectiveness in Elderly Persons Living in the Community

According to the 2013 Cochrane Review on the efficacy and/or effectiveness of influenza vaccines in elderly people in the community, a meta-analysis of data from RCTs and observational studies showed a vaccine efficacy and/or effectiveness of about 49% (95%CI: 33–62%) for laboratory-confirmed influenza and 39% (95%CI: 35–43%) for influenza-like illness [15].

In recent years, case-control study using a test-negative design (TND) has been established to avoid the bias of health-seeking behavior. Influenza vaccine effectiveness in the elderly has been evaluated by using this study design in the past decade. Case-control studies with TND can be adapted for diseases for which patients visit medical institutions immediately after onset and are also used internationally as a standard procedure for monitoring the effectiveness of influenza vaccines. These studies are designed to test all patients who have attended medical institutions with influenza-like illness during the epidemic period and to compare the vaccination rates of the two groups with tests that yield positive results for cases and negative results for controls [16]. A systematic review and meta-analysis using 56 case-control studies with TND (January 1, 2004 to March 31, 2015) showed that pooled vaccine effectiveness against influenza was 33% (95%CI: 26–39%) for A(H3N2), 54% (95%CI: 46–61%) for type B, 61% (95%CI: 57–65%) for A(H1N1)pdm09, and 67% (95%CI: 29–85%) for A(H1N1). Vaccine effectiveness against influenza type A(H3N2) was lower than that for other virus types, and such association was evident in the elderly [17]. Another meta-analysis of 35 case-control studies with TND reported that seasonal influenza vaccine was not significantly effective during local virus activity, irrespective of vaccine match or mismatch to the circulating virus strain. During sporadic virus activity, vaccine effectiveness against laboratory-confirmed influenza was significant only when the vaccine strain matched the circulating virus strain (vaccine effectiveness: 31%; 95%CI: 1–52%). During virus regional activity or widespread activity, influenza vaccine was significantly effective irrespective of vaccine strain match or mismatch to the circulating virus strain, and the vaccine effectiveness was higher than that during sporadic activity [18]. Vaccine effectiveness during regional season for matched and unmatched strains was 58% (95%CI: 40–70%) and 43% (95%CI: 21–59%), respectively, and that during widespread season was 46% (95%CI: 38–54%) and 28% (95%CI: 15–40%), respectively.

Thus, influenza vaccine effectiveness is influenced by many factors including age and immunological response of the vaccinated individual, degree of matching between the vaccine strain and circulating strain, and outcome measurement.

12.6 Immunogenicity of Influenza Vaccination

Evaluation of influenza vaccine should basically examine vaccine effectiveness against the target outcome. However, it is difficult to examine vaccine effectiveness in the following cases: (1) advanced evaluation of the extent by which the vaccine can protect against influenza, (2) incidence of the target outcome is extremely low, (3) control of a pandemic of a new influenza strain is necessary, and (4) vaccine doses and product must be quickly determined. In such cases, established substitute indicators (surrogate markers) such as antibody titer, which is correlated with protection against disease onset, are used.

In the evaluation of influenza vaccine, serum collected before vaccination and serum sampled 3–4 weeks after vaccination are measured for the antibody titer (HI value) using the hemagglutination inhibition (HAI) test. The following variables are calculated: geometric mean titer for HAI, seroprotection rate (proportion of vaccinated individuals with serum HAI titer $\geq$1:40), seroconversion rate (proportion of subjects with pre-vaccination HAI antibody titer <1:10 and post-vaccination titer HAI $\geq$1:40, or a pre-vaccination titer $\geq$1:10 and a fourfold antibody increase after vaccination), and mean fold rise. The US Food and Drug Administration defines adequate response criteria as follows: the lower limit of the two-sided 95%CI for the seroprotection rate is $\geq$60% or that for seroconversion rate is $\geq$30% (Table 12.1) [19]. According to the European Medicines Evaluation Agency crite-

Table 12.1 Immunogenicity response for the licensure of seasonal inactivated influenza vaccines

US Department of Health and Human Services and Food and Drug Administration
For adults <65 years of age and for the pediatric population:
• The lower bound of the two-sided 95% CI for the percentage of subjects achieving seroconversion for HI antibody should meet or exceed 40%
• The lower bound of the two-sided 95% CI for the percentage of subjects achieving an HI antibody titer >1:40 should meet or exceed 70%
For adults >65 years of age:
• The lower bound of the two-sided 95% CI for the percentage of subjects achieving seroconversion for HI antibody should meet or exceed 30%
• The lower bound of the two-sided 95% CI for the percentage of subjects achieving an HI antibody titer >1:40 should meet or exceed 60%
European Agency for the Evaluation of Medical Products
For adults between 18 and 60 years of age, at least one of the assessments should meet the indicated requirements:
• Number of seroconversions or significant increase in anti-hemagglutinin antibody titer >40%
• Mean geometric increase >2.5
• Proportion of subjects achieving an HI titer $\geq$40 should be >70%
For adults >60 years of age, at least one of the assessments should meet the indicated requirements:
• Number of seroconversions or significant increase in anti-hemagglutinin antibody titer >30%
• Mean geometric increase >2.0
• Proportion of subjects achieving an HI titer $\geq$40 should be >60%

ria for evaluating HAI antibody responses to a seasonal vaccine, a seroprotection rate >60%, a seroconversion rate >30%, or a mean geometric increase >2.0 is considered the cut-off values for vaccine immunogenicity in adults 18–60 years of age (Table 12.1) [20].

Although the seroprotection level, defined as HAI titer ≥40, is considered to be associated with approximately 50% clinical protection from infection, this standard was established in young healthy adults. Thus far, few data suggest that such antibody titers correlate with protection among the elderly. Conversely, to our knowledge, no study has reported on the minimal HI titer to indicate protection against infection, and neither seroprotection nor seroconversion predicts infection. However, HAI antibody titer is presently used as a serological marker for protection from influenza.

Most studies suggest that antibody responses to influenza vaccination are decreased in the elderly. It is probable that increased immune system dysregulation with aging contributes to the increased likelihood of serious complications of influenza infection. According to a review of 31 studies of immunogenicity against seasonal influenza vaccine, seroprotection and seroconversion rates of elderly persons were significantly lower than those of healthy adults [21]. The current split vaccine has low immunogenicity especially in the elderly, which is one of the factors of low influenza vaccine effectiveness in such individuals. The need for improvement of immune response and vaccine effectiveness among adults ≥65 years of age has led to the development and licensure of vaccines intended to promote a better immune response in this population. In the USA, adjuvanted, high-dose, live attenuated, and genetically modified vaccines have been approved and used [22].

12.7 Safety of Influenza Vaccine

The most frequent side effect of vaccination was soreness at the vaccination site that lasted <2 days. These local reactions were mild and rarely interfered with the recipients' ability to conduct usual daily activities. In addition, the frequency of side effects in the elderly is reported to be the same as that in adults [23].

12.8 Influenza and Pneumococcal Combination Vaccine

The causative agent of pneumonia during the influenza epidemic period is primarily *S. pneumoniae*, and in death related to the 2009 pandemic, pneumococcal involvement accounted for about 40% of the cases [24]. Therefore, an influenza and pneumococcal combination vaccine may be useful for prevention of pneumonia following influenza in the elderly. This combination vaccine has been reported to significantly reduce hospitalization and death compared with single vaccination [25].

12.9   Conclusions

In this chapter, the characteristics of influenza virus, influenza disease burden in the elderly, and influenza vaccine as an influenza countermeasure and its effectiveness were discussed. Seasonal influenza is a major problem as a cause of complications for the elderly, such as serious pneumonia and related deaths, and it repeatedly circulates annually. The influenza vaccine shows a protective effect against the onset and severity of influenza in elderly people; however, because of its low immunogenicity, it does not reach sufficiently high vaccine effectiveness. In the future, development and introduction of highly immunogenic vaccines are expected. The effectiveness of such influenza vaccines should be evaluated using appropriate epidemiological methods.

References

1. American Academy of Pediatrics. Influenza. In: Kimberlin DW, Brady MT, Jackson MA, Long SS, editors. Red Book: 2015 Report of the committee on infectious diseases. 30th ed. Elk Grove Village, IL: American Academy of Pediatrics; 2015. p. 476–93.
2. Yu X, Tsibane T, McGraw PA, House FS, Keefer CJ, Hicar MD, et al. Neutralizing antibodies derived from the B cells of 1918 influenza pandemic survivors. Nature. 2008;455(7212):532–6.
3. Hancock K, Veguilla V, Lu X, Zhong W, Butler EN, Sun H, et al. Cross-reactive antibody responses to the 2009 pandemic H1N1 influenza virus. N Engl J Med. 2009;361(20):1945–52.
4. Itoh Y, Shinya K, Kiso M, Watanabe T, Sakoda Y, Hatta M, et al. In vitro and in vivo characterization of new swine-origin H1N1 influenza viruses. Nature. 2009;460(7258):1021–5.
5. National Institute of Infectious Diseases Japan. Influenza in this season (2016/17) in Japan. 2017 (in Japanese). https://www.niid.go.jp/niid/images/idsc/disease/influ/fludoco1617.pdf.
6. Reed C, Chaves SS, Daily Kirley P, Emerson R, Aragon D, Hancock EB, et al. Estimating influenza disease burden from population-based surveillance data in the United States. PLoS One. 2015;10(3):e0118369.
7. Holter JC, Muller F, Bjorang O, Samdal HH, Marthinsen JB, Jenum PA, et al. Etiology of community-acquired pneumonia and diagnostic yields of microbiological methods: a 3-year prospective study in Norway. BMC Infect Dis. 2015;15:64.
8. Hirota Y, Kaji M. History of influenza vaccination programs in Japan. Vaccine. 2008;26(50):6451–4.
9. Reichert TA, Sugaya N, Fedson DS, Glezen WP, Simonsen L, Tashiro M. The Japanese experience with vaccinating schoolchildren against influenza. N Engl J Med. 2001;344(12):889–96.
10. Fiore AE, Uyeki TM, Broder K, Finelli L, Euler GL, Singleton JA, et al. Prevention and control of influenza with vaccines: recommendations of the Advisory Committee on Immunization Practices (ACIP), 2010. MMWR Recomm Rep. 2010;59(RR-8):1–62.
11. Nobuhara H, Watanabe Y, Miura Y. Estimation of influenza vaccination coverage in Japan (in Japanese). Jpn J Public Health. 2014;61(7):354–9.
12. Greenwood M, Yule GU. The statistics of anti-typhoid and anti-cholera inoculations, and the interpretation of such statistics in general. Proc R Soc Med. 1915;8(Sect Epidemiol State Med):113–94.
13. Harper SA, Fukuda K, Uyeki TM, Cox NJ, Bridges CB. Prevention and control of influenza. Recommendations of the Advisory Committee on Immunization Practices (ACIP). MMWR Recomm Rep. 2005;54(RR-8):1–40.

14. Hara M, Sakamoto T, Tanaka K. Effectiveness of influenza vaccination in preventing influenza-like illness among community-dwelling elderly: population-based cohort study in Japan. Vaccine. 2006;24(27–28):5546–51.
15. Beyer WE, McElhaney J, Smith DJ, Monto AS, Nguyen-Van-Tam JS, Osterhaus AD. Cochrane re-arranged: support for policies to vaccinate elderly people against influenza. Vaccine. 2013;31(50):6030–3.
16. Fukushima W, Hirota Y. Basic principles of test-negative design in evaluating influenza vaccine effectiveness. Vaccine. 2017;35(36):4796–800.
17. Belongia EA, Simpson MD, King JP, Sundaram ME, Kelley NS, Osterholm MT, et al. Variable influenza vaccine effectiveness by subtype: a systematic review and meta-analysis of test-negative design studies. Lancet Infect Dis. 2016;16(8):942–51.
18. Darvishian M, Bijlsma MJ, Hak E, van den Heuvel ER. Effectiveness of seasonal influenza vaccine in community-dwelling elderly people: a meta-analysis of test-negative design case-control studies. Lancet Infect Dis. 2014;14(12):1228–39.
19. Center for Biologics Evaluation and Research. Guidance for industry: clinical data needed to support the licensure of pandemic influenza vaccines. Bethesda, MD: Food and Drug Administration; 2007. https://www.fda.gov/BiologicsBloodVaccines/GuidanceCompliance RegulatoryInformation/Guidances/Vaccines/ucm074794.htm.
20. European Committee for Proprietary Medial Products. Note for guidance on harmonisation of requirements for influenza vaccine (CPMP/BWP/214/96). London: European Agency for the Evaluation of Medical Products; 1997. http://www.ema.europa.eu/pdfs/human/bwp/021496en.pdf.
21. Goodwin K, Viboud C, Simonsen L. Antibody response to influenza vaccination in the elderly: a quantitative review. Vaccine. 2006;24(8):1159–69.
22. Grohskopf LA, Sokolow LZ, Broder KR, Walter EB, Bresee JS, Fry AM, et al. Prevention and control of seasonal influenza with vaccines: recommendations of the Advisory Committee on Immunization Practices—United States, 2017–18 influenza season. MMWR Recomm Rep. 2017;66(2):1–20.
23. Govaert TM, Dinant GJ, Aretz K, Masurel N, Sprenger MJ, Knottnerus JA. Adverse reactions to influenza vaccine in elderly people: randomised double blind placebo controlled trial. BMJ. 1993;307(6910):988–90.
24. Centers for Disease Control and Prevention. Bacterial coinfections in lung tissue specimens from fatal cases of 2009 pandemic influenza A (H1N1)—United States, May–August 2009. MMWR Morb Mortal Wkly Rep. 2009;58(38):1071–4.
25. Christenson B, Lundbergh P, Hedlund J, Ortqvist A. Effects of a large-scale intervention with influenza and 23-valent pneumococcal vaccines in adults aged 65 years or older: a prospective study. Lancet. 2001;357(9261):1008–11.

Chapter 13
The Great East Japan Earthquake, the Fukushima Daiichi Nuclear Power Plant Accident, and Elderly Health

Seiji Yasumura

Abstract On March 11, 2011, Japan experienced an earthquake of magnitude 9-9.1, called the Great East Japan Earthquake, with a subsequent giant tsunami, which caused massive damage to the Tohoku region Pacific coast (Iwate, Miyagi, and Fukushima prefectures), and a nuclear accident that occurred at the Fukushima Daiichi nuclear power plant. Disaster-related deaths occurred mainly in the elderly, and more than half of the disaster-related deaths occurred in Fukushima prefecture, where the nuclear accident occurred. During the first 2 years after the Great East Japan Earthquake, the suicide standard mortality ratio (SMR) in the three affected prefectures decreased. Three years after the disaster, however, the suicide SMR rose to the pre-disaster level in Iwate and Miyagi prefectures and exceeded the suicide SMR before the disaster in Fukushima prefecture. Mental health service providers for disasters should keep in mind that suicide rates can eventually increase after a disaster, even if they initially decrease.

Keywords Great East Japan Earthquake · A nuclear accident at a nuclear power plant · Suicide · Elderly

13.1 Introduction

13.1.1 Demographic Characteristics of Japan: Aging Society

Since World War II, the population of Japan has been aging at a very rapid rate compared with rates in European countries. The period from the time that the aging proportion [1] of the population was more than 7% (an "aging society") to the period when there was an aging proportion of 14% or more (an "aged society") was

S. Yasumura
Department of Public Health, Fukushima Medical University School of Medicine, Fukushima City, Fukushima, Japan
e-mail: yasumura@fmu.ac.jp

© Springer Nature Singapore Pte Ltd. 2019
M. Washio, C. Kiyohara (eds.), *Health Issues and Care System for the Elderly*, Current Topics in Environmental Health and Preventive Medicine, https://doi.org/10.1007/978-981-13-1762-0_13

40 years in Germany, which has the most rapidly aging population in Europe, but this period was only 24 years in Japan [2]. It is clear that the rate of Japan's population aging is extremely fast. Now the proportion of elderly people aged 65 years or older in Japan has reached 27.7% (2017) [3]

The cabinet of Japan has noted two main reasons for the rapid aging of Japan's population [4]. The first reason is that the mortality rate for elderly people (those aged 65 or older) has rapidly declined since World War II. The reasons for this rapid decline include improvements in public health, better nutrient conditions, and the development of medical technology. Especially, the dramatic decline in neonatal and infant mortality has also contributed to the decreasing mortality rate in Japan. And mortality in elderly people of both sexes has decreased gradually in every age group, which means that the older proportion of the population is becoming relatively larger. Another reason for the rapid aging of the population is that the fertility rate has decreased over time. The crude birth rate has decreased from 13.6 (per 1000, in 1980) to 7.8 (per 1000, in 2016) [5]. This means there is a decrease in the extent of the young generation itself, as well as a decrease in the pool of potential mothers who have the possibility of having babies in the future.

Now Japan has become a "super-aged society", where the proportion of the elderly (i.e., those aged 65 years or older) is higher than 21% [1]. The Japanese National Institute of Population [2] has estimated that the proportion of the elderly in the population will be 35.7% in 2050 (Fig. 13.1).

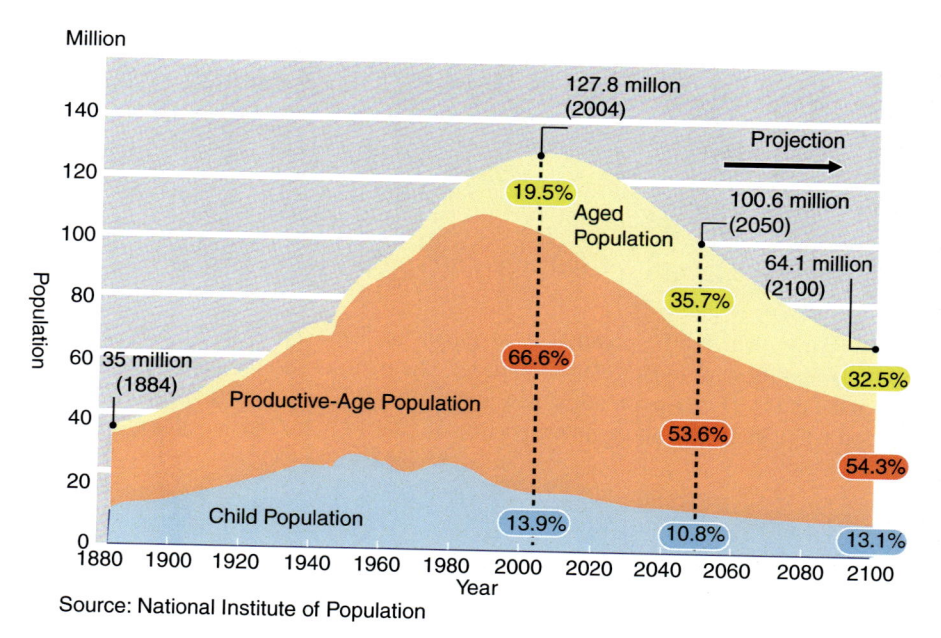

Fig. 13.1 Population trends in Japan [2]

13.1.2 Life Expectancy at Birth and Healthy Life Expectancy at Birth in Japan

Between 1947 and 2016 in Japan, life expectancy at birth increased by 30.92 years for males and by 33.18 years for females, reaching 80.98 years and 87.14 years, respectively, in 2016 [6]. Because life expectancy at birth is calculated by summing the age-adjusted mortality, the lengthening of life expectancy at birth means a decrease in total mortality. The reason for the decrease in the mortality rate is as described above.

Some points should be noted. Life expectancy at birth in males did not increase compared with that in females. Gender differences of life expectancy at birth have, rather, expanded. The true reason is not known, but inappropriate lifestyle factors in males, such as a high smoking rate and a high drinking rate, may have contributed to the gender difference.

In developed countries, life expectancy at birth has increased and this increase has not been so remarkable in recent years. Of note, not all elderly people are healthy and fit; some need nursing care and are bedridden and/or have severe cognitive dysfunction. Healthy life expectancy at birth, which is a new idea, indicates the period during which people can sustain their activities of daily living without receiving nursing care or becoming bedridden.

In Japan, healthy life expectancy at birth in males rose from 69.40 years in 2001 to 70.42 years in 2010; in females, healthy life expectancy at birth rose from 72.65 years in 2001 to 73.62 years in 2010 [7] (Fig. 13.2). The difference between life expectancy at birth and healthy life expectancy at birth in males was 8.67 years in 2001 and this figure had increased to 9.13 years in 2010; on the other hand, the difference between life expectancy at birth and healthy life expectancy at birth in females was 12.28 years in 2001 and this had increased to 12.68 years in 2010. The important point is that the gap between life expectancy at birth and healthy life expectancy at birth did not decrease, but rather expanded in both sexes. Reducing the gap is a big issue to be solved.

13.1.3 Increasing survivorship in the elderly population in Japan

The number of survivors of a certain age in a certain year is calculated as the accumulation of age-specific mortality up to that age. A high mortality rate means poor health, while a low mortality rate means good health. Therefore, the fact that the number of survivors is small implies that the mortality rate is high; that is, the health condition is poor, whereas a high number of survivors implies that the mortality rate is low; that is, the health condition is good. The Japan life tables for 1947, 1955, 1975, 2010, and 2015, showing female survivors who reach a specific age, are displayed in Fig. 13.3 [8].

Survivorship curves can be drawn using only the mortality rate data at each age in a certain year by sex. It can be seen, in Fig. 13.3, that the survivorship

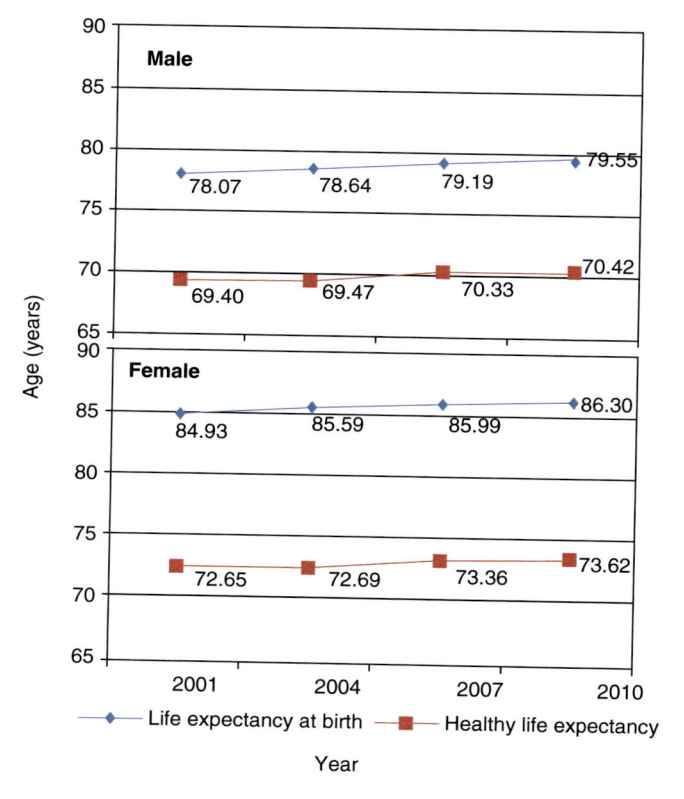

Fig. 13.2 Life expectancy at birth and healthy life expectancy by sex [7]

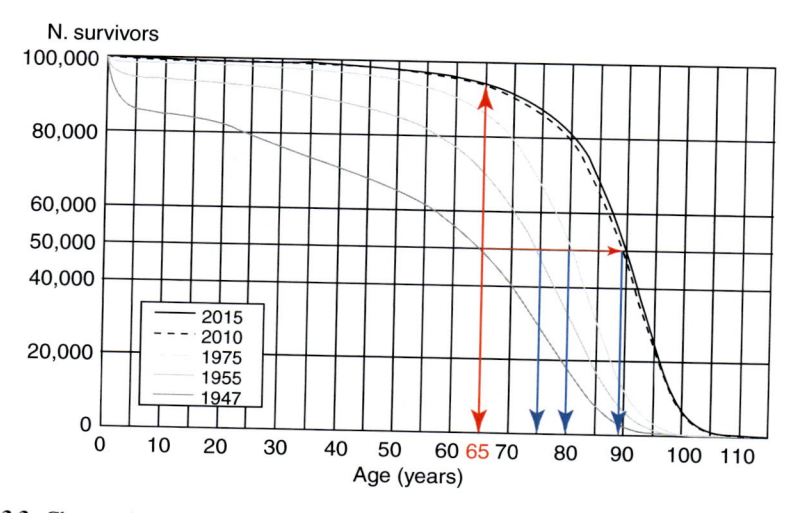

Fig. 13.3 Changes in numbers of survivors (female) [8]

curve has shifted to the right with time, which means that the number of survivors at each age increased in all age groups. The number of the young to middle-aged group increased from 1947 to 1955; on the other hand, that of the elderly group showed a relative increase from 1975 to 2015. Immediately after World War II, improvements in health levels in young to middle-aged people were remarkable, and from 1975 onward, improvements in health conditions have been remarkable in elderly people.

We can see that about half of the female babies born in 1947 (50,000/100,000) lived to be 65 years old. For example, ages at the time that about half of these babies lived to be 65 years old were about 75 years, 80 years, and 88 years in 1955, 1975, and 2010, respectively. This finding means that elderly Japanese females have tended to survive for longer over this period (1955 to 2010), which indicates that elderly Japanese females have become fitter over time. The same tendency was observed in Japanese males (data not shown). These data show that elderly people in Japan have continued to become healthier in both sexes.

13.1.4 Physical, Psychological, and Social Aspects of the Elderly Population in Japan

Various data on the physical and psychological health of the elderly population in recent years in Japan has shown that, in the current group of elderly people, the changes in physical function accompanying aging are delayed by 5–10 years as compared with data from 10–20 years ago [9]. There is a so-called "rejuvenation" phenomenon. Even in those aged 65 years or older, who have been regarded as elderly, especially those at the ages of 65–74, physical and mental health is being maintained, and the majority of those who are capable of active social activities are so occupied.

In regard to social aspects, according to the labor force survey conducted by Japanese Government, in 2016 the labor force participation rate for the elderly population (aged over 65 years) was 31.7% for males and 15.9% for females, both of which rates have been increasing in recent years [10]. On the other hand, the percentage of the labor force aged between 15 and 24 years is about 44% for both males and females; i.e., this group represents less than half the labor force. Thus, it is not appropriate to regard people aged 15–64 years as the "productive-age population." This term was used when the majority of Japanese did not go to high school and got a job at age 15 years. It is thought that this term is now inappropriate and there is a concern that it could promote ageism. We need to know that elderly people are not a social burden or a group who always require medical/nursing care services and pensions, but that some elderly people also contribute to society through their labor.

Under these circumstances, the working group focusing on the definition and classification of "elderly" in the Japan Gerontological Society and the Japan Geriatrics Society have made the following proposal [9]. They have proposed that the definition of "elderly" needs to be changed, with those aged 65–74 years defined as "pre-old people," those aged 75–89 years as "old people," and those aged over 90 as "oldest old people" or "superold elderly."

There are some concerns regarding the change in definition of the elderly. Some people think that the national government wants the elderly to keep working to compensate for the nation's labor shortage, so these people worry about whether this proposal will be implemented. They are also worried that the age at which a pension payment starts may be increased as the definition of elderly changes.

In the Japan Cabinet Office's "survey on the consciousness of elderly people," the percentage of people who regard the elderly as those "from the age of 70", which was the most frequent answer, was 29.1%. The second most common answer was "from the age of 75," at 27.9%. The consciousness of what constitutes an "elderly" population has also changed year by year [11]. We need to consider various possibilities of defining what is regarded as elderly.

13.2 The Great East Japan Earthquake, the Fukushima Daiichi Nuclear Power Plant Accident, and the Health of the Elderly

13.2.1 The Elderly in a Disaster Situation

We need to consider how elderly people are regarded in the context of a disaster situation. As mentioned above, the elderly population varies greatly in its physical, psychological, and social aspects.

In general, elderly people can be regarded as belonging to one of the following three categories: (1) independent and frail elderly living in their homes without a care service, (2) elderly people who use a care service in their homes, and (3) elderly people who live in institutions for the elderly or who are hospitalized because of chronic diseases. The number of people who belong to the latter two categories represents a relatively small proportion of the total elderly population but a relatively large proportion of the total population.

"People requiring assistance during a disaster," as defined by the Cabinet office, Government of Japan et al., refers to those who need help to take necessary actions in the case of a disaster [12]. This includes acquiring accurate and necessary information in a prompt manner and getting evacuated to safer places to protect from the disaster. Generally, this group includes the elderly, disabled people, foreigners, expectant mothers, and young children. The data described in reference [12] shows that elderly people are more susceptible to becoming victims of disaster than young people. Elderly people constitute one of the most vulnerable populations in the case of a disaster [13].

13.2.2   Evacuation Support Plan

The Basic Act on Disaster Control Measures in Japan defines a disaster. The Act requires each municipality to create an evacuation support plan. The plan prescribes the management and duty to, first, collect information, such as that on housing, information transmission systems, and the type of needed care, related to "people requiring assistance during a disaster"; secondly, there is a duty to manage and share the information, using electronic or paper data; and thirdly, there is a duty to select a sufficient number of evacuation supporters for all "people requiring assistance during a disaster." The appropriate securing of an evacuation route is a very big and difficult problem.

In order to create an evacuation support system, the collecting and sharing of information during normal times, not only on "people requiring assistance during a disaster" but also on the total elderly population, is crucial. There are three methods for municipalities to collect and share information. Firstly, using the rule of utilization other than for intended purposes and the provision of data in the municipal Personal Information Protection Regulation, related institutions and members can share information without permission from the elderly individuals. Secondly, after informing people of the creation of an evacuation support system, information only on those who want to register themselves is collected. Thirdly, related institutions and members directly meet the "people requiring assistance during a disaster" and get information from them.

13.2.3   Life and Health Control Guidelines for Evacuation [14]

Once a severe disaster has occurred, people are requested to evacuate to the appropriate shelter or regional evacuation center. According to the guideline for controlling the health condition of people living in the shelter, the shelters are controlled and managed by the municipalities (Table 13.1).

Municipalities also create special shelters, named "welfare shelters", for "people requiring assistance during a disaster". Welfare shelters [15] are secondary evacuation centers that are established for elderly people and people with disabilities who find it difficult to stay at evacuation centers and need special assistance. In accordance with the Disaster Relief Act, municipalities form agreements with various bodies, such as preregistered welfare facilities.

Table 13.1 Guideline for control of the health condition of people living in shelters [14]

	Category	Contents
Daily living; general checkpoint	Living conditions, air and ventilation	1. Temperature control
		2. Maintaining cleanliness of bedclothes, supporting exchange of bedclothes
		3. Control of mosquito, fly, mice, and cockroach
	Water	1. Water replacement to the elderly who don't recognize such condition
		2. Sanitation of water supply
	Nutrition control	Supply good balanced meal based on the required quantity
	Prevention of food poisoning	Sanitation of food regardless of season
	In case of no bathing space	Supply warm towel to evacuees to wipe their own bodies to keep their body clean
	Environment of the surrounding the shelter	1. Make sink and toilet and keep them clean
		2. Collection of garbage, separate and sort them into several types, and storage them in closed space outside the shelter
		3. Decide the rule of drinking alcohol and smoking. Make sure that everyone is informed on the rule to avoid passive smoking and fire. No smoking inside the shelter
Disease prevention and maintenance of good mental health; general checkpoint	1. Prevention of outbreak of infection	2. Prevention of inhalation of dust
	3. Prevention of worsening of chronic diseases	4. Prevention of economy class syndrome
	5. Prevention of disuse syndrome	6. Prevention of heatstroke
	7. Prevention of hypothermia	8. Oral sanitation
	9. Prevention of carbon monoxide poisoning	10. Prevention of worsening of allergic diseases
	11. Health checkup	12. Building emergency consultation system

13.2.4 Great East Japan Earthquake

On March 11, 2011, an earthquake of 9.0–9.1 magnitude, the Great East Japan Earthquake, occurred off the Pacific coast of Tohoku prefecture, and a subsequent giant tsunami hit the coastal area of Japan, especially the northeast area. Many people died and many are still lost. Also, a nuclear accident occurred at the Tokyo Electric Power Company's Fukushima Daiichi nuclear power plant (NPP) and an evacuation zone was designated by the national government, according to the radiation dose in Fukushima, immediately after the accident.

Table 13.2 Number of disaster-related deaths after the Great East Japan Earthquake, by prefecture and age [16]

Prefecture	Total	Age group		
		≤20	>21 <66	≥66
Iwate	446	1	55	390
Miyagi	900	2	113	785
Fukushima	1793	0	169	1624
Others	55	3	10	42
Total	3194	6	347	2841

13.2.4.1 Disaster-Related Deaths

Over 164,000 people in Fukushima were forced to evacuate to areas outside the evacuation zone or they evacuated voluntarily from their living place to other places. In Fukushima, due to earthquakes and/or the tsunami, 1613 people died, and 204 people are still lost, as of September 30, 2017. In addition, 2202 deaths occurred as a result of the Fukushima Daiichi NPP accident (Table 13.2) [16]. These deaths are called "disaster-related deaths." Disaster-related death is defined as death not caused by the direct effect of an earthquake/tsunami but death caused by the worsening of a person's present disease or caused by a new disease that occurred after the disaster. The question we asked is "What type of person has a disaster-related death? Disaster-related deaths occurred mainly among the elderly (aged 66 years or over), while very few people aged 20 years or less died of a disaster-related cause. More than half of the disaster-related deaths after the Great East Japan Earthquake occurred in Fukushima prefecture.

13.2.4.2 Evacuation Stress in Disasters

Another point I would like to emphasize is the severe stress that occurs during evacuation. All inpatients in hospitals and residents in social institutions inside the evacuation zone were forced to evacuate by the government. Figure 13.4 shows changes in mortality rates in the institutionalized elderly before and after the Fukushima NPP accident. The quarterly mortality ratio for the first 3 months after the disaster was 3.1, followed by 1.8 for the next 3 months and 1.4 for another 6 months [17]. This finding, which shows that the negative effects of the evacuation continued for more than 1 year after the disaster, indicates that long-term evacuation was a serious stressor in the elderly residents. We need to take into account the relocation stress in the elderly, regardless of whether the relocation is compulsory or voluntary.

13.2.4.3 Suicide after the Great East Japan Earthquake

It is easy to understand that people who experience a severe disaster may become depressed and/or have post-traumatic stress disorder (PTSD). After the Great East Japan Earthquake, the suicide standardized mortality ratio (SMR) decreased during

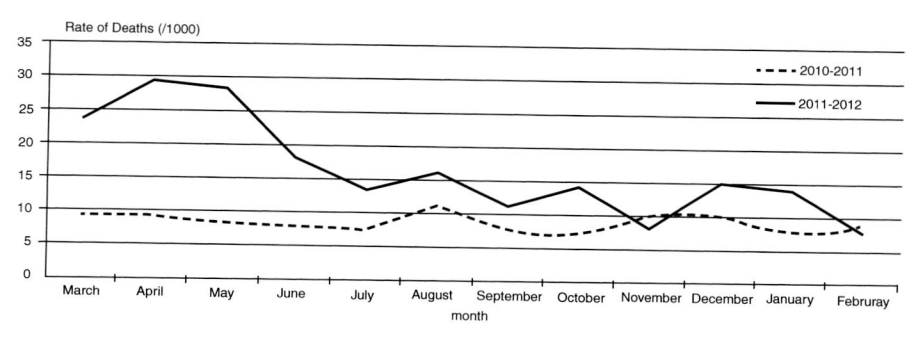

Fig. 13.4 Changes in mortality rates in the institutionalized elderly before and after the Fukushima nuclear power plant accident [17]

the first 2 years in the three affected prefectures (Iwate, Miyagi, and Fukushima) compared with the rates in 2010. The suicide SMR then rose in 2014 to the pre-disaster level in Iwate and Miyagi prefectures, while it exceeded the pre-disaster level in Fukushima prefecture [18]. Five years after the nuclear accident, using monthly data from vital statistics in the evacuation areas in Fukushima between March 2009 and December 2015, analysis by age revealed that post-disaster male suicide rates in the evacuation areas had decreased for those aged 50–69 years and had increased for those aged 29 years or less and those 70 years or older [19]. These findings suggest that providers of disaster mental health services need to keep in mind that suicide rates can eventually increase after a disaster, even if they initially decrease.

13.3 Conclusion

In 2011, Japan experienced the Great East Japan Earthquake, a subsequent giant tsunami hit the coastal area, and there was a nuclear accident at Fukushima Daiichi NPP. We need to consider how elderly people are regarded in the context of a disaster situation, as, generally, elderly people are more likely to become victims of a disaster than are young people. For "people requiring assistance during a disaster" accurate and necessary information needs to be acquired in a prompt manner so that these people can be evacuated to safer places to protect them from the disaster.

Disaster-related death is defined as death not caused by a direct effect of an earthquake/tsunami but death caused by worsening of a person's present disease or death caused by a new disease that occurred after the disaster. After the Great East Japan Earthquake, disaster-related deaths occurred mainly in the elderly, and more than half of these deaths occurred in Fukushima prefecture, where the nuclear accident occurred. The quarterly mortality ratio for the first 3 months after the disaster was 3.1, followed by 1.8 for the next 3 months and 1.4 for another 6 months. We also need to take into account the relocation stress of this group, regardless of whether their relocation is compulsory or voluntary.

After the Great East Japan Earthquake, suicide SMRs decreased during the first 2 years in the three affected prefectures (Iwate, Miyagi, and Fukushima) and in 2014 these rates rose to the pre-disaster level in Iwate and Miyagi prefectures and exceeded the pre-disaster level in Fukushima prefecture. Providers of disaster mental health services should keep in mind that suicide rates can eventually increase after a disaster, even if they initially decrease.

References

1. World Health Organization. The uses of epidemiology in the study of the elderly. Report of a WHO Scientific Group on the Epidemiology of Aging. World Health Organ Tech Rep Ser. 1984;706:1–84.
2. National Institute of Population and Social Security Research, Japan. National Institute of Population and Social Security Research Pamphlet. P4. 2017.
3. Statistics Bureau, Ministry of Internal Affairs and Communication, Government of Japan. Population projection. 2017. http://www.stat.go.jp/data/topics/topi1031.html (in Japanese). Accessed 3 Apr 2018.
4. Cabinet Office, Government of Japan. 2017. http://www8.cao.go.jp/kourei/whitepaper/w-2017/zenbun/29pdf_index.html (in Japanese). Accessed 3 Apr 2018.
5. Ministry of Health, Labour and Welfare, Government of Japan. Vital statistics 2017. Ministry of Health, Labor and Welfare (in Japanese).
6. Director-General for Statistics and Information Policy, Ministry of Health, Labour and Welfare, Government of Japan. Abridged life tables for Japan 2016. http://www.mhlw.go.jp/english/database/db-hw/lifetb16/dl/lifetb16-06.pdf. Accessed 3 Apr 2018.
7. Ministry of Health, Labour and Welfare, Government of Japan. p. 2. http://www.mhlw.go.jp/bunya/kenkou/dl/chiiki-gyousei_03_02.pdf (in Japanese). Accessed 3 Apr 2018.
8. Ministry of Health, Labour and Welfare, Government of Japan. The 22nd life tables. p. 6. http://www.mhlw.go.jp/toukei/saikin/hw/life/22th/dl/22th_11.pdf (in Japanese). Accessed 3 Apr 2018.
9. Ouchi Y, Rakugi H, Arai H, Akishita M, Ito H, Toba K, et al. Redefining the elderly as aged 75 years and older: proposal from the Joint Committee of Japan Gerontological Society and the Japan Geriatrics Society. Geriatr Gerontol Int. 2017;17(7):1045–7. https://doi.org/10.1111/ggi.13118.
10. Ministry of Health, Labor and Welfare, Government of Japan. Year Book of Labor Statistics 2017. http://www.stat.go.jp/data/roudou/report/2016/pdf/summary1.pdf (in Japanese). Accessed 3 Apr 2018.
11. The Cabinet, Government of Japan. Survey on the consciousness of elderly people. 2014. http://www8.cao.go.jp/kourei/ishiki/h26/sougou/zentai/pdf/s2-8.pdf (in Japanese). Accessed 3 Apr 2018.
12. The Cabinet, Ministry of Public Management, Ministry of Health, Labor and Welfare, Government of Japan. Guideline for "people requiring assistance during a disaster". 2006. p. 3 (in Japanese).
13. Yasumura S. Support for people requiring assistance during a disaster. In: Yasumura S, Kamiya K, editors. Public health in a nuclear disaster—message from Fukushima. Hiroshima: Hiroshima University Press; 2014. p. 406–8.
14. The Cabinet, Japan. Evacuation life and health control guideline. 2016. p. 4. http://www.bousai.go.jp/taisaku/hinanjo/pdf/1605hinanjo_guideline.pdf (in Japanese). Accessed 3 Apr 2018.
15. The Cabinet, Japan. Evacuation life and health control guideline in welfare shelter. 2016. p. 4. http://www.bousai.go.jp/taisaku/hinanjo/pdf/1604hinanjo_hukushi_guideline.pdf (in Japanese). Accessed 3 Apr 2018.

16. Reconstruction Agency, Government of Japan. Number of disaster-related deaths in Great East Japan Earthquake. http://www.reconstruction.go.jp/topics/main-cat2/sub-cat2-6/20171226_kanrenshi.pdf (in Japanese). Accessed 3 Apr 2018.
17. Yasumura S. Evacuation effect on excess mortality among institutionalized elderly after the Fukushima Daiichi nuclear power plant accident. Fukushima J Med Sci. 2014;60(2):192–5. https://doi.org/10.5387/fms.2014-13.
18. Ohto H, Maeda M, Yabe H, Yasumura S, Bromet EE. Suicide rates in the aftermath of the 2011 earthquake in Japan. Lancet. 2015;385(9979):1727. https://doi.org/10.1016/S0140-6736(15)60890-X.
19. Orui M, Suzuki Y, Maeda M, Yasumura S. Suicide rates in evacuation areas after the Fukushima Daiichi nuclear disaster: a 5-year follow-up study in Fukushima prefecture. Crisis. 2018:1–11. https://doi.org/10.1027/0227-5910/a000509.